KT-562-141

Introduction

We are very pleased that our book has gone into a second edition. Anxiety disorders are common and disabling conditions. Their scientific and medical study has presented numerous problems, stemming partly from diagnostic complexities and partly from issues relating to treatment. We have attempted to provide the medical practitioner and other interested health professionals and lay people with a succinct yet informative introduction to the area.

In this second edition, we have retained and updated almost all of the original content. We have added a section dealing with caffeine and anxiety, and we have taken the opportunity to clarify some of the areas discussed in the first edition.

The most significant developments have been seen in the arena of therapy, in which changes are proceeding apace. The major swing has been away from sedative and tranquilizer medications, and towards antidepressants with a primary action on the serotonin systems. We have therefore updated the drug treatment sections to reflect these advances.

In parallel, psychological treatments have become more focused and effective, and we have outlined the commonly used management strategies.

We hope that the reader will find this revised edition of continuing use, and that it will enable both professional and lay people with an interest in anxiety disorders to obtain a rapid overview of the most important topics.

1 Definitions

Anxiety is a normal part of the response to a challenging or threatening situation. As such, it may actually be advantageous. However, severe, persistent or inappropriate anxiety can impair everyday life, as well as affecting occupational and social functioning. Anxiety symptoms, including palpitations, sweating, trembling and feelings of fear and panic, are a common finding among patients in primary care. Such patients may complain of:

- primary symptoms of nervousness, apprehension, irritability and restless sleep
- a constellation of physical signs and symptoms, particularly in certain situations
- a combination of both.

The distinction between anxiety symptoms and disorders is an important one. In many individuals, symptoms are a normal reaction to everyday problems or major life events, and such patients may not need treatment. In contrast, primary anxiety disorders, in which the anxiety is abnormal in quality or severity, and often inappropriate or unrelated to the external situation, are disabling and lead to significant distress or impairment in work or social functioning. As a result, patients' quality of life is usually adversely affected. Behavioral and pharmacological therapies are required to enable patients to resume a normal life.

This book describes anxiety disorders, psychiatric conditions with particular characteristics, and their management. It covers generalized anxiety, panic disorder, various phobic disorders and related conditions, obsessive–compulsive disorder and post-traumatic stress disorder.

Anxiety disorders

The term 'anxiety disorders' subsumes a number of well-defined conditions in which anxiety is a predominant clinical feature (Table 1.1). They are usually classified according to the American Psychiatric Association's *Diagnostic and Statistical Manual of Mental Disorders*, currently in its fourth edition (DSM-IV), or the World Health Organization's *International Classification of Diseases and Related Health Problems* (ICD-10). Definitions used in this book are based on DSM-IV, though the ICD-10 definitions are essentially similar.

Generalized anxiety disorder (GAD) is the most common anxiety disorder, with an estimated point prevalence of about 3% among both the UK and US adult populations. The prevalence among patients consulting their family physicians is about 15%; hence, this condition makes considerable demands on primary care services.

GAD is characterized by persistent and markedly inappropriate anxiety, with motor tension, autonomic hyperactivity, apprehension and vigilance. Circumstances associated with this excessive apprehension or worry include concerns about health, finances, job performance, marital

TABLE 1.1

Anxiety disorders

- Generalized anxiety disorder
- Panic disorder (with or without agoraphobia)
- Agoraphobia
- Social anxiety disorder
- Specific (simple) phobia
- Obsessive–compulsive disorder
- Acute stress and post-traumatic stress disorders

relationships or other life events. However, individuals with GAD often cannot identify the specific sources of their worry and will complain of fatigue, muscle aches and twitches, trouble swallowing and an inability to control troublesome thoughts.

When the source of worry can be identified, the degree of apprehension about otherwise understandably distressing situations is clearly abnormal, and results in impairment of work or social functioning. When upsetting situations are resolved, they are almost always replaced by another concern, which may be a revisited old worry or an entirely new problem. Patients with GAD seeking treatment typically complain of nearly uninterrupted anxiety and tension for months or years. The DSM-IV criteria for this condition are summarized in Table 1.2.

Other anxiety and mood disorders often occur in association with GAD. In the US National Institute of Mental Health Epidemiological Catchment Area Study, for example, 54% of patients in whom GAD was diagnosed had concomitant panic or depressive illness.

Panic disorder is the most common problem encountered in patients seeking medical help because of mental health problems. Panic disorder is characterized by panic attacks (i.e. circumscribed periods of intense fear or discomfort) associated with physical symptoms such as, but not limited to:
- chest discomfort
- palpitations
- sweating
- shortness of breath
- dizziness
- paresthesias.

TABLE 1.2

DSM-IV criteria for generalized anxiety disorder

- Unrealistic or excessive anxiety and worry (apprehensive expectation) about two or more life circumstances, lasting at least 6 months; the patient is bothered by these concerns on more days than not
- Focus of anxiety and worry is unrelated to any concomitant disorder
- Disturbances do not occur only during the course of mood or psychotic disorders
- At least six of the following symptoms are often present when the patient is anxious (excluding symptoms present only during panic attacks):

Motor tension
- trembling, twitching, feeling shaky
- muscle tension, aches or soreness
- restlessness
- easy fatigability

Autonomic hyperactivity
- shortness of breath or sensations of smothering
- palpitations or tachycardia
- sweating or cold, clammy hands
- dry mouth
- dizziness or light-headedness
- nausea, diarrhea or other abdominal distress
- hot flushes or chills
- frequent urination
- difficulty in swallowing, 'lump in throat'

Vigilance and scanning
- feeling keyed up or on edge
- exaggerated startle response
- difficulty concentrating or 'mind going blank' because of anxiety
- trouble falling or staying asleep
- irritability

- It cannot be established that an organic factor (e.g. hyperthyroidism, caffeine intoxication) initiated or maintained the disturbance

Reprinted with permission from the *Diagnostic and Statistical Manual of Mental Disorders*, fourth edition. Copyright © 2000 American Psychiatric Association.

Because of their severity and sudden onset, panic attacks are often misperceived as being imminently life-threatening by patients (as well as physicians), particularly when the attacks are associated with tachycardia and chest pain. Many patients first present to the Accident and Emergency Departments of general hospitals, convinced they are going to die. Others may fear going mad or losing control of themselves and their bodily functions.

Patients can usually give graphic accounts of their first attack, timing it to the nearest minute. In contrast to phobias (see pages 15–16), panic attacks most typically occur unexpectedly, at least in the initial stages of the disorder; they are not provoked by exposure to a particular stimulus.

Panic disorder can severely impair quality of life, with patients becoming progressively more disabled by the attacks themselves and fear of the attacks, as well as by the secondary development of avoidance behaviors. The DSM-IV criteria for panic disorder are shown in Table 1.3.

Complications. Approximately 65% of panic disorder patients develop agoraphobia. Agoraphobia, like all phobias, can be defined as a persistent and irrational fear of a specific object, activity or situation (a phobic stimulus) that results in a compelling desire to avoid the stimulus. In the case of agoraphobia, which is almost always associated with panic disorder, the person articulates a fear of being in places or situations from which escape might be difficult or impossible in the event of sudden incapacitation. Among the clinically significant phobias, agoraphobia is the most common and disabling.

People with agoraphobia organize their daily activities to make sure that help will be available in case of an emergency. Typically, patients restrict travel away from home or rely on a companion when going out. In mild cases of agoraphobia,

TABLE 1.3

DSM-IV criteria for panic disorder

- Recurrent panic attacks (discrete periods of intense fear or discomfort with abrupt onset) that are uncued (i.e. do not occur immediately before or on exposure to a situation that almost always causes anxiety, and are not triggered by situations in which the person was the focus of others' attention)
- At least one such attack must be followed by at least one of the following:
  - persistent concern about additional attacks
  - worry about the implications of an attack or its consequences (e.g. losing control, having a heart attack, 'going crazy')
  - a significant change in behavior related to the attacks
- At least four of the following symptoms must occur during at least one attack:
  - palpitations
  - pounding heart or accelerated heart rate
  - sweating
  - trembling or shaking
  - sensations of shortness of breath or smothering
  - feeling of choking
  - chest pain or discomfort
  - nausea or abdominal distress
  - feeling dizzy, unsteady, light-headed or faint
  - derealization (loss of sense of reality) or depersonalization
  - fear of losing control or going crazy
  - fear of dying
  - paresthesias
  - chills or hot flushes
- During at least some of the attacks, at least four of the symptoms listed above should reach a peak within 10 minutes of the onset of the first symptom
- It cannot be established that an organic factor (e.g. hyperthyroidism, caffeine intoxication) initiated or maintained the disturbance

Reprinted with permission from the *Diagnostic and Statistical Manual of Mental Disorders*, fourth edition. Copyright © 2000 American Psychiatric Association.

individuals are able to leave home but will avoid specific situations such as crowded places, driving, escalators or elevators. In severe cases, patients may be unable to leave their home or even a particular room in their house. These severely agoraphobic patients must rely on supportive individuals to purchase food and supply other essentials of daily living.

Some specific fears commonly associated with agoraphobia include:

- being in a strange place
- crossing streets
- crowds or crowded places, such as supermarkets
- elevators
- journeys away from home, particularly in underground trains
- open spaces.

Thus, agoraphobia describes various secondary fears that develop as a consequence of panic attacks. Although agoraphobia has been reported to occur in the absence of panic disorder, this is rarely observed in clinical practice. The DSM-IV criteria for agoraphobia without panic disorder are presented in Table 1.4.

Social anxiety disorder is defined as an excessive fear of situations in which the person may be evaluated or scrutinized by others, or an excessive fear of acting in an embarrassing way in such situations. Examples of social anxiety disorders include:

- fear of public speaking or performance
- fear of talking to superiors or peers
- fear of eating in public
- fear of using public lavatories
- fear of dating.

TABLE 1.4

DSM-IV criteria for agoraphobia without panic disorder

- The person must not have previously met the criteria for panic disorder

- The person often fears the occurrence of either panic symptoms or limited symptom attacks (fewer than four symptoms)

- The person may or may not have experienced such attacks previously

- Avoidance of specific situations must not be accounted for by another disorder

Reprinted with permission from the *Diagnostic and Statistical Manual of Mental Disorders*, fourth edition. Copyright © 2000 American Psychiatric Association.

These conditions are distinguished from agoraphobia in that the individual is concerned with avoiding the risk of being observed by others, rather than avoiding the situation itself. Thus, symptoms experienced by a social phobic may increase (or worsen) in the 'observing' presence of a friend, but may reduce (or improve) in an agoraphobic person who is accompanied by a trusted companion.

Social phobics do not, for example, have trouble presenting a speech in private, but will have tremendous difficulty giving the identical speech in public. By contrast, an agoraphobic who has a specific fear of elevators will remain fearful whether using the elevator in private or with a companion. It is true that the agoraphobic may have more courage to do things with the support of a companion, but the focus of the fear has not changed (i.e. he or she remains frightened of going in the elevator). The DSM-IV criteria for social anxiety disorder are shown in Table 1.5.

Specific phobias (previously referred to as simple phobias) are defined as excessive fear of an object or situation, other than those involved in agoraphobia or social anxiety disorder. The most common specific phobias relate to:

- animals (particularly dogs, snakes, insects, spiders, birds or mice)
- blood or injury
- enclosed spaces (claustrophobia)
- heights (acrophobia)
- storms
- dental procedures
- driving
- air travel.

Typically, affected people experience abrupt anxiety symptoms to the point of intense panic-like anxiety on

---

TABLE 1.5

DSM-IV criteria for social anxiety disorder

- Persistent fear of one or more situations in which the person is exposed to public scrutiny by others, and fears that he or she may do something that is, or act in a manner that is, embarrassing or humiliating

- This fear is unrelated to other disorders (e.g. panic attacks, Parkinson's disease or eating disorders)

- During some phase of the disturbance, exposure to the specific stimulus almost invariably provokes an immediate anxiety response

- The phobic situation is avoided or endured with intense anxiety

- Avoidance behavior interferes with occupational or usual social activities, or relationships with others, or there is marked distress about the phobia

- The person recognizes that their fear is excessive or unreasonable

Reprinted with permission from the *Diagnostic and Statistical Manual of Mental Disorders*, fourth edition. Copyright © 2000 American Psychiatric Association.

exposure to the stimulus. They therefore make great efforts to avoid the stimulus. The DSM-IV criteria for specific phobias are shown in Table 1.6.

Obsessive–compulsive disorder (OCD) is characterized by recurrent thoughts or impulses (obsessions) that are recognized as unwanted, irrational or unpleasant, but are nevertheless irresistible (Table 1.7). The response to obsessions consists of repetitive, ritualized acts (compulsions), which occur in up to 75% of people with obsessions. More than one obsession may be present in an individual, but multiple compulsions are rare. OCD is often associated with intense anxiety and intrusive unwanted thoughts, leading to impairment of everyday life.

TABLE 1.6

DSM-IV criteria for specific phobias

- Persistent fear of a circumscribed stimulus (object or situation), other than fear of having a panic attack (as in panic disorder) or of humiliation or embarrassment in certain social situations (as in social anxiety disorder)
- During some phase of the disturbance, exposure to the stimulus almost invariably provokes an intense anxiety response
- The stimulus is avoided or endured with intense anxiety
- The fear or associated avoidance behavior significantly interferes with the person's normal routine, or with usual social activities or relationships with others, or there is marked distress about having the fear
- The person recognizes that their fear is excessive or unreasonable
- The stimulus is unrelated to the content of the obsessions of obsessive–compulsive disorder or post-traumatic stress disorder

Reprinted with permission from the *Diagnostic and Statistical Manual of Mental Disorders*, fourth edition. Copyright © 2000 American Psychiatric Association.

TABLE 1.7

DSM-IV criteria for obsessive–compulsive disorder

A Either obsessions or compulsions

Obsessions

1 Recurrent and persistent thoughts, impulses or images that are experienced, at some time during the disturbance, as intrusive and inappropriate and that cause marked anxiety or distress

2 The thoughts, impulses or images are not simply excessive worries about real-life problems

3 The person attempts to ignore or suppress such thoughts, impulses or images, or to neutralize them with some other thought or action

4 The person recognizes that the obsessional thoughts, impulses or images are a product of his or her own mind (not imposed from without, as in thought insertion)

Compulsions

1 Repetitive behaviors (e.g. hand washing) or mental acts (e.g. counting) that the person feels driven to perform in response to an obsession, or according to rules that must be applied rigidly

2 The behaviors or mental acts are aimed at preventing or reducing distress, or preventing some dreaded event or situation; however, these behaviors or mental acts are either not connected in a realistic way with what they are designed to neutralize or prevent, or are clearly excessive

B At some point during the course of the disorder, the person has recognized that the obsessions or compulsions are excessive or unreasonable

C The obsessions or compulsions cause marked distress, are time-consuming (take more than 1 hour a day) or significantly interfere with the person's normal routine, occupational (or academic) functioning, or usual social activities or relationships

Reprinted with permission from the *Diagnostic and Statistical Manual of Mental Disorders*, fourth edition. Copyright © 2000 American Psychiatric Association.

Post-traumatic stress disorder (PTSD) is defined in DSM-IV as a reaction to exposure to traumatic events involving actual or threatened death or serious injury, or a threat to the physical integrity of oneself or others, with a response of intense fear, helplessness or horror. The most common causes of PTSD are combat, rape or other violent crime, and natural and manmade disasters (e.g. plane crashes). DSM-IV criteria for PTSD are summarized in Table 1.8. Symptoms include:

- feelings of guilt
- autonomic and sleep disturbances
- difficulty in concentrating
- irritability and aggressiveness
- intrusive thoughts
- 'flashbacks'.

These symptoms can lead to a full panic attack in response to cues that trigger memories of the traumatic event.

Anxiety as a symptom of concomitant illness

Psychiatric illness. Anxiety symptoms may be associated with a number of other psychiatric conditions. In particular, anxiety is a common concomitant finding with depressive disorders.* About 60% of depressed patients are diagnosed with an anxiety disorder, and many patients with an apparent primary anxiety disorder develop depression over time. Schizophrenia is commonly associated with anxiety symptoms, but the absence of psychotic symptoms such as delusions or hallucinations distinguishes the anxiety disorders from schizophrenia. However, severe anxiety or panic attacks may be the presenting symptoms of an incipient psychotic breakdown. Substance abuse, particularly with amphetamines and cocaine, can lead to severe anxiety symptoms.

*See the second edition of *Fast Facts: Depression*, by David S Baldwin and Robert MA Hirschfeld, published by Health Press Limited in 2005.

TABLE 1.8

DSM-IV criteria for post-traumatic stress disorder

A The person has been exposed to a traumatic event in which both of the following were present:

  1 The person experienced, witnessed or was confronted with an event or events that involved actual or threatened death or serious injury, or a threat to the physical integrity of self or others

  2 The person's response involved intense fear, helplessness or horror

  Note: In children this response may be expressed instead by disorganized or agitated behavior

B The traumatic event is persistently re-experienced in one (or more) of the following ways:

  1 Recurrent and intrusive distressing recollections of the event, including images, thoughts or perceptions

  2 Recurrent distressing dreams of the event

  3 Acting or feeling as if the traumatic event were recurring

  4 Intense psychological distress at exposure to internal or external cues that symbolize or resemble an aspect of the traumatic event

  5 Physiological reactivity on exposure to internal or external cues that symbolize or resemble an aspect of the traumatic event

C Persistent avoidance of stimuli associated with the trauma and numbing of general responsiveness (not present before the trauma)

D Persistent symptoms of increased arousal (not present before the trauma), as indicated by two (or more) of the following:

  1 Difficulty in falling or staying asleep

  2 Irritability or outbursts of anger

  3 Difficulty in concentrating

  4 Hypervigilance

  5 Exaggerated startle response

E Duration of the disturbance (symptoms in criteria B, C and D) is more than 1 month

F The disturbance causes clinically significant distress or impairment in social, occupational or other important areas of functioning

Reprinted with permission from the *Diagnostic and Statistical Manual of Mental Disorders*, fourth edition. Copyright © 2000 American Psychiatric Association.

Medical conditions. Various medical conditions are associated with anxiety (Table 1.9). It is not surprising that concern about illness and medical treatment may itself provoke anxiety. However, some conditions may produce intrinsic symptoms that resemble or mimic primary anxiety disorders. Thyrotoxicosis is often associated with anxiety and may closely resemble either GAD or panic disorder.

Key points – definitions

- It is important to distinguish anxiety symptoms that are a normal reaction to everyday problems or major life events from those associated with anxiety disorders. Treatment may not be required if anxiety levels are appropriate to the situation.
- Anxiety disorders are disabling, impair patients' work and social functioning, and require psychological or pharmacological intervention.
- Generalized anxiety disorder is the most common anxiety disorder, with a point prevalence of 3% in the primary care population.
- About two-thirds of patients who have panic disorder develop agoraphobia.
- Anxiety is a common concomitant finding with depressive disorders. About 60% of depressed patients are also diagnosed with an anxiety disorder, and many patients who have a primary anxiety disorder develop depression.
- Misuse of cocaine, amphetamines and 'ecstasy' has led to an increase in severe anxiety symptoms in adolescents and young adults.

TABLE 1.9

Medical conditions associated with anxiety symptoms

Drug-related

Intoxication

- anticholinergic drugs
- xanthines (caffeine, theophylline)
- steroids
- amphetamines, cocaine
- aspirin
- hallucinogens
- sympathomimetic agents
- tobacco

Withdrawal

- alcohol
- sedatives/hypnotics
- narcotics

Cardiovascular/respiratory

Hypoxia

Congestive heart failure

Mitral valve prolapse

Pulmonary embolism

Cardiac dysrhythmias

Hypertension

Myocardial infarction or angina

Endocrine

Carcinoid syndrome

Hyperparathyroidism

Menopausal symptoms

Pituitary disorders

Cushing's syndrome

Hyperthyroidism

Pheochromocytoma

Premenstrual syndrome

Neurological and other disorders

Anaphylaxis

Huntington's disease

Multiple sclerosis

Pain

Ulcerative colitis

Wilson's disease

Epilepsy

Migraine

Organic brain syndrome

Peptic ulcer

Vestibular dysfunction

Drug-related events (intoxication or withdrawal) are probably the most common causes of secondary anxiety in patients with medical conditions. The increase in misuse of stimulant drugs such as cocaine, amphetamines and 'ecstasy' has led to an increase in the number of reports of anxiety symptoms, often severe, in adolescent and young adult populations. In addition, cardiovascular and respiratory conditions can also provoke anxiety due to:

- feelings of shortness of breath
- awareness of cardiac function (e.g. tachycardia)
- pain associated with cardiac disease
- fear associated with the illness.

Mitral valve prolapse has been reported to be associated with anxiety, although there is evidence that prolapse in anxious patients tends to be mild and clinically insignificant.

Key reference

American Psychiatric Association Task Force on DSM-IV. *Diagnostic and Statistical Manual of Mental Disorders: DSM-IV*. Washington, DC: American Psychiatric Association, 1994.

Genetic factors

Several lines of evidence indicate that genetic factors play a role in the anxiety disorders, though non-biological factors, psychosocial stressors, conditioning and learning are also relevant in the etiology of pathological anxiety states.

• Studies of patients with panic disorder reveal that 18% of first-degree relatives (i.e. parents, offspring, siblings) have the same disorder, compared with 2% of more distant relatives. In addition, 60% of patients have at least one relative with the same disorder, compared with 15% of control patients.

• The concordance rate in studies in twins (i.e. the proportion of cases in which a condition occurs in both members of a pair of twins) has been reported to be 45% in identical twins, compared with 15% in non-identical twins.

• First-degree relatives of patients seeking treatment for specific phobias have been shown to be more likely to have a specific phobia than family members of patients without phobias. Furthermore, studies in twins have consistently shown a greater concordance of specific phobias in identical than in non-identical twins.

Theories of anxiety

A number of biological and psychological theories have been proposed to describe the origins and mechanisms of anxiety disorders. In general, these focus on abnormalities in neurotransmitter function and psychological disturbances, particularly involving cognition (Table 2.1).

TABLE 2.1

Theories to explain the development of anxiety disorders

Physiological

Abnormal neurotransmitter/neuromodulator function

- norepinephrine (noradrenaline)
- 5-hydroxytryptamine (5-HT, serotonin)
- γ-aminobutyric acid (GABA)
- adenosine
- cholecystokinin

Psychological

Psychoanalytical theories

Learning theories

Abnormal neurotransmission/neuromodulation. Several abnormalities in neurotransmitter or neuromodulatory systems have been implicated in the pathogenesis of anxiety disorders, notably norepinephrine, serotonin (5-hydroxytryptamine; 5-HT), adenosine, cholecystokinin (CCK) and γ-aminobutyric acid (GABA). Neurosteroids may also play a role.

Norepinephrine. Increased activity of the noradrenergic (norepinephrine) system has been suggested as a factor in the development of panic attacks. Evidence for this theory comes from observations in animal and clinical studies.

- Anxiety can be provoked by activation of the noradrenergic system.
- Plasma and cerebrospinal fluid concentrations of norepinephrine and its metabolite 3-methoxy-4-hydroxy-phenylglycol (MHPG) are increased in the presence of anxiety.
- The α_2-adrenergic antagonist yohimbine provokes more anxiety and panic, and a greater increase in MHPG

concentrations, in patients with panic disorder than in patients without the condition.

Serotonin. The activity of the serotonergic system also appears to be increased in anxiety. This is thought to be due to enhanced sensitivity at postsynaptic 5-HT receptors. Evidence that the serotonergic system is involved in anxiety comes from a number of observations.

- Benzodiazepines, which are effective anxiolytic agents (see page 66), decrease 5-HT turnover in serotonergic neurons.
- Treatment with *m*-chlorophenylpiperazine (*m*CPP), a 5-HT agonist, increases anxiety.
- The selective serotonin-reuptake inhibitors (SSRIs) are effective in the treatment of panic anxiety (see page 71), but can actually increase anxiety in the first few days of administration.

γ-Aminobutyric acid. The GABA theory suggests that anxiety is due to a decrease in the inhibitory activity of GABA-containing neurons. Thus benzodiazepines, which act at GABA receptors, are believed to act by enhancing this inhibition.

Adenosine. Decreased activity or function of adenosine has been implicated in anxiety. Evidence suggesting that adenosine may modulate systems of anxiety or fear is as follows.

- Adenosine is an endogenous substance with natural anticonvulsant properties.
- Adenosine produces sedation and lowers heart rate in animals.
- Caffeine blocks adenosine receptors.
- Caffeine and stress independently upregulate brain adenosine receptors.
- Caffeine augments the effects of stress in humans and animals.

- Acute and chronic caffeine intoxication mimic panic disorder and generalized anxiety disorder, respectively, in humans.
- Caffeine stimulates panic attacks and produces high blood cortisol and lactate levels in panic-prone people.

While adenosine neuromodulation appears to be involved in the biochemistry of anxiety, it is notable that agents with blocking actions at adenosine receptors also influence other receptor systems implicated in the biochemistry of anxiety, namely GABAergic and noradrenergic systems.

Cholecystokinin. Disturbances in CCK function have been suggested as a possible factor in many different forms of anxiety. The following observations support this theory.

- CCK concentrations are lower in the cerebrospinal fluid of patients with panic disorder.
- Cholecystokinin-tetrapeptide (CCK-4), a smaller molecular form of CCK, produces panic attacks and more severe anxiety in patients with panic disorder than in normal control subjects.
- Pentagastrin, a 5-amino-acid peptide that incorporates the 4-amino-acid sequence of CCK-4, produces significantly greater anxiety or panic attacks in patients with panic disorder, social anxiety disorder or obsessive–compulsive disorder than in normal controls.
- Anxiety-producing effects of CCK-4 are blocked in humans by CCK receptor antagonists that preferentially bind to the CCK receptor subtype (CCK-B) that is most prominent in the brain.

It is possible that new CCK-B antagonist drugs with anxiolytic actions may be developed in the future.

Multiple interactions. Clearly, the biochemical basis of anxiety is complex, and it is likely that multiple interactions between the adenosinergic, noradrenergic, serotonergic and

> **Key points – pathophysiology of anxiety**
>
> - Genetic factors, non-biological factors, psychosocial stressors, conditioning and learning all play a role in anxiety disorders.
> - Norepinephrine, serotonin, adenosine, cholecystokinin and γ-aminobutyric acid may be implicated in the pathogenesis of anxiety disorders; neurosteroids may also play a role.
> - Behavioral and cognitive therapies are based on the concept that anxiety can be learned and unlearned through experience.

GABAergic systems are involved. For example, the serotonergic and GABAergic systems are closely related, both functionally and anatomically, and hence facilitation of GABA activity by benzodiazepines could indirectly reduce the activity of the serotonergic system. Similarly, the anxiety-provoking effects of the noradrenergic system may be modulated by the serotonergic system.

Psychological theories of anxiety include psychoanalytical and learning theories.

Psychoanalytical theories. It has been suggested that anxiety results when the ego is overwhelmed by excitation from the outside world, from the id (unconscious instincts) or from the superego (a part of the mind acting as a check on the id – in effect, as a conscience). Psychoanalytical theories have much less influence now than hitherto.

Learning theories. It has been postulated that anxiety is a fear response that has been attached to another stimulus by conditioning. Thus, anxiety can be learned and unlearned through experience; this is the basis of behavioral and cognitive therapies for anxiety (see Chapter 6, pages 60–5).

Key references

McCann UD, Slate SO, Geraci M et al. A comparison of the effects of intravenous pentagastrin on patients with social phobia, panic disorder and healthy controls. *Neuropsychopharmacology* 1997;16:229–37.

Siegel GJ, Agranoff BW, Albers RW et al. *Basic Neurochemistry: Molecular, Cellular and Medical Aspects*. Philadelphia: Lippincott, Williams & Wilkins, 1998.

Uhde TW, Singareddy R. Biological research in anxiety disorders. In: Maj M, ed. *Psychiatry as a Neuroscience*. New York: John Wiley and Sons, 2002:237–85.

Uhde TW, Tancer ME, Rubinow DR et al. Evidence for hypothalamo–growth hormone dysfunction in panic disorder: profile of growth hormone (GH) responses to clonidine, yohimbine, caffeine, glucose, GRF and TRH in panic disorder patients versus healthy volunteers. *Neuropsychopharmacology* 1992;6:101–18.

Yehuda R. Biology of post-traumatic stress disorder. *J Clin Psychiatry* 2000;61(suppl 7): 14–21.

Anxiety disorders are common in primary care patients, but are often unrecognized and untreated; their exact prevalence remains to be determined. Most information on the epidemiology of these disorders comes from the US National Comorbidity Survey (NCS), which used the diagnostic criteria presented in the revised third edition of the DSM (the DSM-IV criteria are very similar). In general, this survey has found higher prevalences for most anxiety disorders than those reported in the earlier Epidemiological Catchment Area (ECA) study. The different estimates of prevalence reflect differences in the criteria for being regarded as a medical case (i.e. requiring treatment), together with variations in interviewing techniques and sampling frameworks.

Survey results

The prevalence estimates for the most common anxiety disorders reported in the NCS are shown in Table 3.1. This study suggests that, overall, almost one quarter of the population will experience an anxiety disorder during their lifetime. In contrast, the ECA study estimated that the lifetime prevalence was 14.6% and the 6-month prevalence was 8.9%. In both studies, anxiety disorders were more common than mood disorders (mainly depression). The NCS data also suggest that social and specific phobias are the most common phobias. The prevalence of these phobias was considerably higher than that reported in the ECA study (6-month prevalence of 1.2% and lifetime prevalence of 2.2% for social anxiety disorder, and 4.5% and 11.8%, respectively, for specific phobias).

TABLE 3.1

Prevalence of anxiety disorders in the National Comorbidity Survey

	Lifetime (%)	12-month (%)
Generalized anxiety disorder	5.1	3.1
Panic disorder	3.5	2.3
Agoraphobia (without panic disorder)	5.3	2.8
Social anxiety disorder	13.3	7.9
Specific phobia	11.3	8.8
Any anxiety disorder	24.9	17.2

Relatively little information is available about the prevalence of obsessive–compulsive disorder (OCD). Obsessive or compulsive symptoms, or both, occur in about 14% of the general population, but the prevalence of true OCD is considerably lower. It is estimated that about 3% of the population will be affected at some time during their lives.

Post-traumatic stress disorder (PTSD) is estimated to have a lifetime prevalence of about 1% in the general population. However, by definition this condition specifically affects people who have been exposed to an extremely traumatic situation or event, hence markedly higher prevalences are seen among such individuals. In a study of US Vietnam war veterans, for example, the lifetime prevalence of PTSD was estimated at 30.9% in men and 26.9% in women.

Age and sex. With the exception of conditions that develop during childhood or adolescence, such as school phobia, the prevalence of anxiety disorders is highest in individuals aged 25–34 years, and declines progressively with increasing age. The prevalence is higher in women than in men, sometimes by as much as 2:1.

Key points – prevalence

- Anxiety disorders are common in the primary care population, but are often unrecognized and therefore untreated.
- As many as one in four people may experience an anxiety disorder at some time in their life, according to data from the US National Comorbidity Survey.
- The prevalence of most anxiety disorders is highest in individuals aged 25–34 years, and declines progressively with increasing age.
- Some specific phobias such as school phobia develop in childhood or adolescence.
- The prevalence of anxiety disorders is higher in women than in men, sometimes by as much as 2:1.

Key references

Bienvenu OJ, Samuels JF, Riddle MA et al. The relationship of obsessive–compulsive disorder to possible spectrum disorders: results from a family study. *Biol Psychiatry* 2000;48:287–93.

Kessler RC, Andrade LH, Bijl RV et al. The effects of co-morbidity on the onset and persistence of generalized anxiety disorder in the ICPE surveys. International Consortium in Psychiatric Epidemiology. *Psychol Med* 2002;32:1213–25.

Kurlan R, Como PG, Miller B et al. The behavioral spectrum of tic disorders: a community-based study. *Neurology* 2002;59: 414–20.

Maier W, Falkai P. The epidemiology of comorbidity between depression, anxiety disorders and somatic diseases. *Int Clin Psychopharmacol* 1999;14(suppl 2):S1–6.

The clinical presentations of the various anxiety disorders differ. In each case, the disorder may resemble other psychiatric or medical conditions (see Chapter 1). Therefore, a careful differential diagnosis is essential.

Generalized anxiety disorder

Generalized anxiety disorder (GAD) can occur at any age, but the average age at onset is about 21 years. The condition is characterized by undue apprehension or worry lasting for at least 6 months. A variety of psychological and somatic symptoms may be present (Table 4.1). Physical symptoms resulting from anxiety may themselves cause further anxiety, thus setting up a 'vicious circle' (Figure 4.1). GAD is about twice as common in women as in men.

Many patients with GAD report that they have been anxious all their lives, but that symptoms are exacerbated by stressful events. In others, the onset of GAD is associated with identifiable stressors; the severity of the condition is often determined by the number and severity of such stressors. GAD usually persists for several years, with the severity of symptoms fluctuating over time, and depressive features may gradually become more apparent. Epidemiological studies suggest that GAD is usually seen in association with other conditions. In the US National Comorbidity Survey, for example, lifetime and 1-month comorbidity rates were 90% and 66%, respectively. The most common concomitant conditions were dysthymia (chronic mild depression), panic disorder and major depression.

TABLE 4.1

Symptoms of generalized anxiety disorder

Psychological	Physical
Feeling keyed up or on edge	Palpitations
Restlessness	Symptoms of hyperventilation
Difficulty concentrating	– tightness in the chest
Difficulty relaxing	– light-headedness
Exaggerated startle response	– numbness or tingling
	Sweating
	Dry mouth
	Nausea
	Diarrhea
	Frequent urination
	Muscular tension, particularly across the shoulders and back
	Trembling
	Headaches

Differential diagnosis of GAD includes a number of physical and psychiatric conditions, although most are uncommon (see Table 1.9, page 21). The most frequently encountered conditions resembling GAD are hyperthyroidism, alcohol- and drug-related conditions including caffeinism, and some psychiatric conditions.

Symptoms of hyperthyroidism include palpitations, insomnia, sweating and diarrhea. The diagnosis can be confirmed by thyroid function tests.

A number of substances can produce symptoms of anxiety:

• alcohol
• nicotine

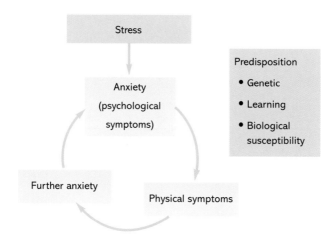

Figure 4.1 The 'vicious circle' of generalized anxiety disorder. Anxiety can produce physical symptoms such as trembling, palpitations, hyperventilation or sweating, which may themselves provoke further anxiety.

- amphetamines
- antihistamines
- slimming tablets
- indometacin
- thyroid preparations
- xanthine compounds (theophylline and caffeine).

Caffeinism is the most commonly unrecognized 'impersonator' of substance-induced generalized anxiety. Caffeine intoxication can mimic both GAD and panic disorder. When the symptoms mimic GAD, the person has typically consumed larger and larger amounts of caffeine, sometimes unsuspectingly, over several weeks or months. While an individual may initially have consumed caffeine to combat fatigue, unintentional consumption of toxic levels may occur through frequent use of over-the-counter medications or beverages not known by the consumer to contain caffeine (see Appendix, pages 85–90).

Initial episodes of stimulant-induced anxiety usually disappear when the substance is discontinued. The exception is individuals at increased genetic risk (i.e. those with first-degree relatives who suffer from GAD), who may still suffer from anxiety after the discontinuation of caffeine or other stimulants. Individuals who are physiologically dependent on caffeine require gradual tapering of their caffeine intake.

Conversely, anxiety symptoms can result from withdrawal of alcohol or other substances, including caffeine. Anxiety is a poorly appreciated but common consequence of caffeine withdrawal in individuals with a history of high caffeine consumption. GAD may therefore be caused both by chronic caffeinism and by caffeine withdrawal.

GAD can occur in association with other psychiatric disorders, notably depression and other mood disorders, other anxiety disorders and early on in schizophrenia.

Panic disorder

Panic attacks take the form of sudden periods of intense anxiety and autonomic arousal. Most occur spontaneously, but attacks may also be provoked by strong emotion, excitement or physical exertion. The anxiety is accompanied by a sense of impending doom, or a feeling that a dreadful event is about to happen. Sufferers fear loss of control (e.g. fainting, urinating or crying out), serious illness or going mad. Between attacks, most patients experience generalized anxiety to some extent. The condition most commonly develops between the ages of 18 and 25 years, and is about two to three times more common in women than in men.

Panic disorder is usually a chronic condition with a fluctuating course, although some patients experience remissions or exacerbations. The relationship between stress and major life events and the severity and course of panic disorder is highly individualized. In some cases, the frequency of panic attacks and severity of agoraphobia parallel the level of life stress. In most cases, however, there appears to be no relationship between severity of illness and life stressors. For example, the death of a spouse or companion has been found to trigger depression, but has little or no impact on the frequency or severity of panic attacks or agoraphobia in patients with a pre-existing diagnosis of panic disorder.

Depression and alcohol abuse are common complications of panic disorder, affecting about 50% and 20% of patients, respectively. Depression develops at some point in the life course of many patients with panic disorder; however, the severity is unpredictable and can range from mild to severe.

Differential diagnosis. A number of cardiovascular, endocrine, neurological and psychiatric conditions are associated with symptoms resembling panic attacks.

Chest pain, breathlessness and palpitations may be precipitated by exercise or emotion in patients with angina. These symptoms can also be caused by cardiac dysrhythmias such as paroxysmal atrial tachycardia; in this case, the diagnosis can be confirmed by electrocardiographic monitoring during an attack.

Anxiety symptoms, including muscle cramps and paresthesias, can occur in some patients with hypoparathyroidism. The presence of carpopedal spasm is a useful diagnostic sign, and the diagnosis can be confirmed by measurement of serum calcium and phosphorus.

In epileptic patients, partial complex seizures may be accompanied by ictal fear and are identical in quality to panic attacks. As shown in Table 4.2, panic attacks are associated with many symptoms mistakenly thought to be pathognomonic of temporal lobe epilepsy. The total number

TABLE 4.2

Psychosensory symptoms in patients with panic disorders

Symptom	Affected patients (%)
Distortion of light intensity	59
Distortion of sound intensity	46
Derealization	46
Strange rising feeling in stomach	41
Depersonalization	37
Sensation of floating, turning, moving	32
Speeding up of thoughts	22
Slowing down of thoughts	20
Jamais vu sensation	17

of psychosensory–psychomotor symptoms experienced during panic attacks is also not significantly different from complex seizures documented by electroencephalography (EEG). The differential diagnosis of panic attacks is also complicated by the fact that patients with complex partial seizures, particularly if untreated for long periods of time, may also develop agoraphobia and similar avoidance behaviors to those observed in patients with panic disorder. Sleep panic attacks and partial seizures are both triggered by sleep deprivation and both have peak occurrences within the first few hours of sleep onset.

From a symptomatic perspective, only the occurrence of fecal or urinary incontinence, loss of consciousness or true tonic–clonic generalizations distinguishes seizures from panic attacks. Gustatory and tactile hallucinations may occur in both disorders, but are associated more often with seizures than wake or sleep panic attacks. EEG recordings can usually establish the appropriate diagnosis. Some patients with panic disorder who fail to respond to traditional antipanic agents (e.g. selective serotonin-reuptake inhibitors) may benefit from anticonvulsant therapy.

Acute caffeine intoxication may mimic panic attacks. Unlike chronic caffeinism, which may imitate generalized anxiety, caffeine-induced panic attacks characteristically develop after the ingestion of large amounts of caffeine (at least 720 mg above the individual's usual daily consumption) in a short period of time. A common scenario is students or truck drivers self-medicating with caffeine to remain awake for prolonged periods.

While large single doses of caffeine (greater than 750 mg) may trigger panic-like symptoms in healthy people, patients with panic disorder are extraordinarily sensitive to caffeine. A dose as low as 100 mg (approximately equivalent to one cup of coffee) may induce severe generalized anxiety or panic attacks. As a consequence of this intrinsic biological vulnerability, most patients with panic disorder learn early in life to avoid caffeinated beverages, foods and medications. This natural sensitivity and tendency to avoid caffeine is not an attribute of individuals with other anxiety disorders.

Approximately 65% of patients who have panic attacks while awake also report nocturnal or sleep panic attacks. Sleep panic attacks typically occur within the first 3 hours of sleep onset, achieve peak intensity within 8 minutes and take place during the transition from late stage 2 to early stage 3 sleep. Symptoms of wake and sleep panic attacks are identical in quality and severity, with the possible exception that a higher proportion of sleep panic attacks may be associated with dyspnea. Sleep panic attacks are not associated with rapid eye movement (REM) sleep, the stage of sleep most often associated with cognitions and vivid imagery.

Like individuals with wake panic attacks, people with sleep panic attacks often develop secondary fears and avoidance behaviors. Thus, sleep panickers develop conditioned fears of sleep environments (e.g. the bedroom) and sleeping itself. Many individuals, particularly men, are embarrassed about their fears and will not freely offer information about sleep phobia. Physicians should therefore ask anxious patients directly about fears relating to sleep.

If untreated, patients with sleep panic attacks may develop chronic sleep deprivation. In addition to the well-documented problems associated with sleep deprivation, such as increased automobile accidents, sleep deprivation markedly worsens symptoms of anxiety and induces panic attacks in patients with panic disorder (Figure 4.2).

Panic attacks can occur in association with mood disorders or other anxiety disorders. For example, about 20% of patients with major depression also have panic attacks. Panic disorder can be distinguished from phobias as the attacks are

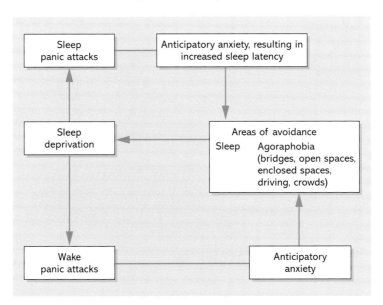

Figure 4.2 Sleep deprivation increases the risk of both sleep and wake panic attacks in patients with panic disorder.

not related to an identifiable stimulus. Panic attacks in patients with GAD can be distinguished from panic disorder, as the attacks in GAD are linked to stressful situations or excessive worry and are not usually as well defined.

Agoraphobia without panic disorder

Although included in DSM-IV, some observers (including the authors) doubt that agoraphobia without panic disorder exists in clinical practice. The criteria are avoidance of situations from which escape might be difficult, or in which help might not be available if anxiety symptoms occur, in people who have never met the criteria for panic disorder. Some investigators supporting the existence of such a syndrome argue that these patients typically fear the occurrence of symptoms of panic attacks, but have not previously experienced such attacks.

Social anxiety disorder

The characteristic feature of social anxiety disorder that can help to confirm the diagnosis is the development of anxiety on exposure to a stimulus. The stimulus may be a single situation or a well-defined set of situations; in most cases, more than one situation is involved (generalized social anxiety disorder).

Performance phobia is a form of social anxiety disorder seen among public performers (e.g. actors and musicians). Situations that may be feared include:
- public speaking
- assertive interactions
- dating
- group activities
- activities that do not involve others, such as eating in public
- performing in public.

Patients show symptoms of autonomic arousal and even panic when exposed to such situations. They worry in anticipation of the situation and anxiously analyze their actions afterwards. The phobia can lead to excessive worry, similar to that seen in GAD; the two conditions are distinguished by the specific relationship of the worry to the social situation.

Social anxiety disorder often develops in late childhood and may present almost exclusively as blushing, shyness and social inhibition. While most blushing and shy children never develop full-blown social anxiety disorder, many adults with the disorder report a long history of these problems, beginning in adolescence or childhood. Selective mutism in very young children is thought by some experts to be a childhood variant of social anxiety disorder. The prevalence of social anxiety disorder is similar in men and women.

If untreated, social anxiety disorder is chronic and unremitting. Some patients manage to avoid the feared situation by lifestyle changes or restrictions. However, the phobic stimulus may sometimes be so extensive that everyday life is severely curtailed. Educational and occupational handicaps may be marked. Alcohol and drug abuse, depression and attempted suicide are common in patients with social anxiety disorder.

Criticism has been leveled by some lay groups, and taken up by the media, that social anxiety disorder is a pseudo-diagnosis. They claim that it is merely medicalizing shyness and is part of the attempt by the medical profession to include normal personality variations within mental diseases. The pronounced functional disabilities, as well as the severe symptomatic distress, suffered by individuals diagnosed as having social anxiety disorder negate these assertions.

41

Specific phobias

Patients with specific phobias usually fear a single object or situation. An amazing number of stimuli can cause phobic reactions that cause distress and, in the authors' experience, include such exotica as the number 13, caviar and canvas.

Some specific phobias are recognized as separate conditions. For example, body dysmorphic disorder is a condition in which the individual believes that they have an abnormality of a body part. They may seek quite unnecessary plastic surgery.

Exposure to the specific feared stimulus produces a strong sense of dread, which may be accompanied by a desire to flee. This may result in strong symptoms of autonomic arousal, including a rise in heart rate and blood pressure, which may become so severe as to resemble panic attacks. Patients with blood phobia have a characteristic reaction, with a sudden decrease in blood pressure leading to dizziness and fainting.

In contrast to GAD and panic disorder, specific phobias usually develop in childhood or adolescence. One study reported that animal phobias develop at an average age of 7 years, blood phobias at an average age of 9 years and dental phobias at an average age of 12 years. Claustrophobia develops at an average age of 20 years.

Little is known about the course of untreated specific phobias. In most cases, the impact of the phobia can be minimized by adopting an appropriate lifestyle to avoid the stimulus. Phobias that develop during childhood are more likely to resolve with time than those that develop later in life.

Differential diagnosis of specific phobias is mainly concerned with distinguishing these conditions from other anxiety disorders. Although the symptoms of specific phobias may resemble panic attacks, they have a specific relationship to the phobic stimulus. By contrast, in panic disorder, symptoms can arise in the absence of a specific stimulus, although particular stimuli may become associated with fear and arousal through conditioning. Illness phobia is difficult to distinguish from hypochondriasis, which is a more wide-ranging preoccupation with illness.

Obsessive–compulsive disorder

The cardinal features of obsessive–compulsive disorder (OCD) are obsessions and compulsions. Patients with OCD report intrusive thoughts, urges or images. Typically, these thoughts or images are characterized as foolish, absurd, stupid, reckless, embarrassing, scandalous or crazy. The person recognizes that these thoughts are irrational, but cannot stop them. Obsessions can, however, take the form of extraordinarily frightening urges (e.g. the impulse to murder a beloved spouse or the notion that you have already injured another person).

Compulsions are repetitive but deliberate acts performed in an attempt to neutralize distressing obsessions. As with obsessions, most people comprehend the irrational nature of their compulsions (e.g. hand washing), and develop continual strategies to resist the urge to perform these acts.

Tics are frequently observed in OCD, and obsessions and compulsions are common problems in patients with Tourette's syndrome and related tic disorders. Body dysmorphic disorder and pathological grooming habits (e.g. nail biting, trichotillomania or skin picking) are found at a higher prevalence in the families of patients with OCD than in the general population.

OCD often develops during childhood, and the prevalence appears to be similar in men and women. Four major obsessions are commonly seen (Table 4.3).

TABLE 4.3

Common presentations of obsessive–compulsive disorder

Obsession	Compulsion
Contamination	Washing
Pathological doubt	Checking
Pure obsession, with intrusive thoughts or urges	Absent (i.e. obsession but no compulsive behavior)
Primary obsessional slowness	

Contamination. The most common obsession is with contamination, which is seen in about 50% of cases. This obsession is usually focused on contamination with bodily products such as urine, feces or vaginal secretions. Patients may spend hours each day washing their hands or bathing; they may also try to avoid possible sources of contamination, but this is not usually successful.

Pathological doubt leads to compulsive checking and rechecking. The patient may fear that lights or fires have been left on and therefore will repeatedly check electric switches or gas taps. This checking, far from resolving the doubt, may actually contribute to further doubt.

Pure obsession, with repetitive, intrusive urges or thoughts, is seen in about 25% of patients with OCD. These thoughts are usually sexual or aggressive in nature, and may be associated with impulses or fearful images.

Primary obsessional slowness is a rare but disabling condition. Such patients may take an hour to brush their teeth, or several hours to eat a meal. Although rituals may be extensive and severe obsessions may be present, such patients show very little anxiety.

Differential diagnosis. The distinction from other anxiety disorders is usually obvious but depression is a common coexistent condition. Early schizophrenia may have an obsessive flavor to some of the symptoms, but the thought content is often peculiar or even bizarre. Obsessional symptoms are occasionally observed in organic cerebral diseases such as encephalitis or streptococcal infections, or after head injury. Although this is highly speculative, observations of obsessive–compulsive-like symptoms in patients with Sydenham's chorea suggest a possible autoimmune basis for early-onset OCD.

The term 'pediatric autoimmune neuropsychiatric disorder associated with streptococcal infections' (PANDAS) has been fashioned to identify individuals whose OCD symptoms appear to have been triggered by group A beta-hemolytic streptococcal (GABHS) infections. PANDAS may also present with tics, attention problems and hyperactivity. While the association between streptococcal infections and OCD is not yet confirmed, it is possible that penicillin prophylaxis might play a future role in the management of patients with OCD or tics in whom PANDAS is suspected.

Post-traumatic stress disorder
Patients with post-traumatic stress disorder (PTSD) may show a variety of symptoms, many of which are shared with other anxiety disorders or depression. Anger, sensations of being ill at ease (dysphoria), and emotional blunting or lability are often present. Diagnostic features include:
- reliving the traumatic event, feeling as if the event is unfolding around them (the patient has some recognition

---

Key points – clinical features

- Generalized anxiety disorder (GAD) is usually seen in association with other disorders, such as depression and panic disorder.
- Hyperthyroidism, alcohol abuse and drug-related conditions, including caffeinism, must be considered in the differential diagnosis of GAD.
- The differential diagnoses of panic disorder include angina, cardiac dysrhythmias, hypoparathyroidism, epilepsy and acute caffeine intoxication.
- Debriefing after a traumatic experience may predispose individuals to developing post-traumatic stress disorder, rather than protect them from it.

---

that the current experience is not real, but rather is a 're-experiencing phenomenon')
- flashbacks, with vivid perceptions of elements of the traumatic event (in these dissociative experiences, the patient believes and behaves as if the event is taking place in reality and at that moment)
- nightmares of the traumatic event
- intrusive recollections of the traumatic event (less vivid than flashbacks or reliving the event, and involving thoughts rather than perceptions).

Sleep disturbances and impaired concentration and memory may also occur. Patients with PTSD usually show chronically increased arousal, but may also react specifically to stimuli that recall the traumatic event, such as loud noises or screams.

PTSD usually develops soon after the traumatic event in the form of an acute condition in which extreme distress, disorientation or dissociation may occur. Repeated severe trauma, such as in combat situations, tends to produce more severe symptoms, which are more likely to occur concomitantly with other disorders and are less likely to resolve without intervention.

Depression, other anxiety disorders and substance abuse are common complications of PTSD. Patients who experience PTSD have high rates of somatic complaints, even in comparison with individuals with panic disorder or GAD. In fact, a diagnosis of PTSD is a stronger clinical predictor of medical complaints such as back pain and arthritis than a history of physical injury or depression. It is unknown whether the increased number of subjective complaints reflects an actual greater prevalence of medical disorders confirmed by laboratory tests.

Although it is common for individuals exposed to severely traumatic events to develop an acute stress reaction, only a minority progress to full PTSD. Recently, it has become evident that debriefing after a stressful experience may predispose some individuals to develop PTSD, rather than protect them from it.

Key references

Mellman TA, Uhde TW. Patients with frequent sleep panic: clinical findings and response to medication treatment. *J Clin Psychiatry* 1990;51:513–16.

Swedo SE, Leonard HL, Garvey M et al. Pediatric autoimmune neuropsychiatric disorders associated with streptococcal infections: clinical description of the first 50 cases. *Am J Psychiatry* 1998;155:264–71.

Uhde TW. Caffeine-induced anxiety: an ideal chemical model of panic disorder. In: Asnis GM, van Praag HM, eds. *Einstein Monograph Series in Psychiatry.* New York: Wiley–Liss, 1995: 181–205.

A variety of psychological and pharmacological therapies can be used in the management of anxiety disorders. In general, most conditions are best managed by a judicious combination of the two approaches.

Psychological therapies

Psychological therapies include:

- counseling
- behavioral therapy, in which patients are taught to tolerate exposure to an anxiety-provoking stimulus
- cognitive therapy, in which patients are taught to recognize the origin and significance of their symptoms, and the role of fearful sensations in maintaining symptoms
- relaxation techniques, biofeedback and meditation
- social skills training.
  These techniques are described in Chapter 6.

Pharmacological therapies

Five principal groups of drugs are used in the management of anxiety disorders:

- benzodiazepines
- selective serotonin-reuptake inhibitors (SSRIs)
- monoamine oxidase (MAO) inhibitors
- tricyclic antidepressants
- buspirone (a 5-HT_{1A} receptor partial agonist).

In addition, β-blockers are still used in the UK, but less so elsewhere. The use of pharmacological therapy is discussed in Chapter 7.

Management plans

Different combinations of psychological and pharmacological therapies are appropriate for each of the anxiety disorders (Table 5.1).

TABLE 5.1

Management techniques for anxiety disorders

	Psychological	Pharmacological
Generalized anxiety disorder	Counseling Relaxation Cognitive therapy	Benzodiazepines Antidepressants Buspirone β-blockers
Panic disorder	Behavioral therapy Cognitive therapy	SSRIs Benzodiazepines Tricyclic antidepressants MAO inhibitors
Agoraphobia	Behavioral therapy	As for panic disorder
Social anxiety disorder	Behavioral therapy Cognitive therapy Social skills training	SSRIs Benzodiazepines β-blockers MAO inhibitors
Specific phobia	Behavioral therapy Cognitive therapy	Not proven to be useful, other than for symptom relief
Obsessive–compulsive disorder	Behavioral therapy	SSRIs Clomipramine
Post-traumatic stress disorder	Crisis intervention Behavioral therapy Cognitive therapy	SSRIs Tricyclic antidepressants MAO inhibitors

MAO, monoamine oxidase; SSRIs, selective serotonin-reuptake inhibitors.

Generalized anxiety disorder (GAD). The first step towards successful management of GAD is identifying the problem. Patients with coexisting depression and anxiety tend to be identified and treated by primary care physicians, but those with pure GAD uncomplicated by depression often go unrecognized. However, even when GAD is unaccompanied by depression, high rates of social and work impairment are seen.

Even if recognized, patients with pure GAD tend to be inadequately treated for their condition. This is unfortunate because many patients with pure GAD can be managed effectively by counseling and, if necessary, other psychological therapies. A series of, for example, four or five consultations over several weeks will often clarify the cause of anxiety and allow the patient to recognize their own role in controlling the condition. Patients with more severe anxiety or those who do not respond to counseling alone may benefit from behavioral therapy and support from the family physician or practice nurse, or from community psychiatric services. Relaxation therapies may also be useful.

For patients who do not respond to psychological treatment alone, a short course of medication may help to control their symptoms. The choice of drug depends on the needs of the individual patient.

- Benzodiazepines are the agents of first choice if a rapid anxiolytic response is required.
- Antidepressants are appropriate for patients with concomitant depression. Several trials have shown venlafaxine to be effective in both the short term (8 weeks) and the long term (6 months). Some SSRIs have also shown efficacy in this indication.
- Buspirone is suitable for the short-term management of anxiety if a quick response is not required. However, the efficacy of buspirone has been questioned.

- β-blockers are often useful in patients in whom mild physical symptoms, such as palpitations, predominate.

Patients who do not respond to primary care treatment should be referred for specialist assessment. Few such patients require hospitalization; most are treated as outpatients, with the continuing involvement of the primary care team.

A working party in the UK has presented guidelines for the management of GAD (Figure 5.1). These guidelines recognize four stages in treatment; however, these stages are not regarded as sequential and treatments from stages 2 to 4 can be combined as appropriate.

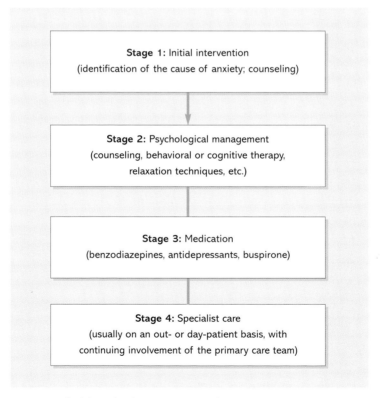

Figure 5.1 Guidelines for the management of generalized anxiety disorder. Treatments listed under stages 2–4 can be combined as appropriate.

Panic disorder. Drug therapy should be considered in all but the mildest cases of panic disorder. The aim of such treatment is to control symptoms, rather than provide permanent relief; relapse is common after stopping treatment. The most effective drugs are:

- SSRIs
- benzodiazepines
- tricyclic antidepressants
- MAO inhibitors.

Behavioral therapy may also be useful in patients with panic disorder, although it plays a lesser role than in patients with phobias. Cognitive therapy may be useful in patients with panic disorder without agoraphobia. In this approach, patients are taught to evaluate and reinterpret sensations that trigger anxiety attacks (e.g. palpitations or light-headedness). They are also taught about the origin of such symptoms, and the role of fear in maintaining them. Relaxation techniques may be helpful as an adjunctive treatment for some patients, but the physician should be aware that relaxation therapy may exacerbate symptoms in those individuals with sleep panic attacks.

Agoraphobia without panic disorder. In the authors' experience, the pure form of this disorder (i.e. agoraphobia without any history of panic attacks) is not seen in clinical practice. There are individuals who report having experienced one or two physical symptoms of discomfort (e.g. sweating, choking sensations, diarrhea), who later worry about or avoid situations that might trigger these symptoms. Such patients may respond to behavioral therapy alone, but a subgroup will ultimately require drug treatment as an adjunct to behavioral therapy in order to achieve a complete response.

In its simplest form, behavioral therapy consists of instructing the patient to expose themselves to phobic situations gradually. The patient should be referred to an anxiety specialist trained in the use of behavioral techniques. The specialist will suggest coping strategies to help the patient face the feared situations.

Social anxiety disorder responds well to both psychological therapy and drug treatment. Behavioral therapy, in which the patient is exposed to the feared stimulus, is of benefit in most cases. Cognitive therapy is also useful.

Four main classes of drugs have been shown to be effective in the management of social anxiety disorder:
- SSRIs and venlafaxine
- benzodiazepines
- β-blockers
- MAO inhibitors.

β-blockers may be effective in performance phobia when physical symptoms of anxiety, such as palpitations, trembling or sweating, are predominant. Otherwise, there is good evidence to support the use of MAO inhibitors, such as phenelzine, or in Europe, the selective reversible MAO inhibitor moclobemide. The efficacy of SSRIs such as paroxetine is also well established and has led to licensing in several countries.

Specific phobias. The behavioral therapy known as systematic desensitization is one of the most effective treatments for specific phobias. Patients learn a muscle relaxation technique and then rank a series of phobic situations according to the amount of anxiety provoked. They expose themselves to the least frightening situation and attempt to relax. Once they are able to relax in this situation, they progress to the next most frightening, and continue this process until the entire range of stimuli has been confronted. Direct exposure to the stimulus (in vivo desensitization) is most effective, but the technique can also be used with images of the phobic stimulus.

Cognitive therapy may be a useful adjunct to desensitization. This allows exaggerated or irrational fears of vulnerability to be addressed, and can also reduce anticipatory anxiety and hypervigilance before potential exposure to a stimulus.

Drug treatment has not been shown to be useful in the management of specific phobias, other than for relief of symptoms. Benzodiazepine treatment at the start of behavioral therapy may be useful in reducing severe anxiety. However, the use of drug treatment during desensitization therapy reduces the effectiveness of the technique, since desensitization relies on the patient experiencing tolerable levels of anxiety. SSRIs and tricyclic antidepressants may be useful in patients with illness phobia, in whom exposure to the stimulus is not possible.

Obsessive–compulsive disorder (OCD). Pharmacotherapy and psychosocial treatments have been found to be effective in the treatment of OCD. However, approximately 50% of patients have an incomplete or unsatisfactory response to standard drug and/or psychological interventions.

Behavioral therapy, with response prevention and distraction techniques, is the most effective form of treatment for OCD. These techniques involve either preventing the patient from carrying out the obsessions, or exposing them, to saturation point, to environmental cues that increase the obsessions. Behavioral therapies may be used alone or in conjunction with medications.

The most effective medications are agents that produce changes in the serotonergic neurotransmitter system (e.g. clomipramine, fluoxetine, fluvoxamine). However, not all serotonergic agents have been shown to be beneficial.

Sleep disturbances are common in OCD, particularly in patients with checking or washing rituals. The selection of a drug to treat obsessions or compulsions should take into account the relative sedating versus activating properties of the agent. Clomipramine tends to be sedating, whereas fluoxetine and fluvoxamine may worsen insomnia. In patients with insomnia, fluoxetine and fluvoxamine should be started at very low doses and increased slowly, as tolerated. Although there is as yet limited evidence to support its use, low doses of trazodone (i.e. 50–100 mg) have been used to counteract the insomnia associated with fluoxetine pharmacotherapy.

Atypical antipsychotics (e.g. quetiapine, risperidone) may also be required, in combination with SSRIs, to achieve a satisfactory response. In patients with partial responses to oral clomipramine, intravenous administration has been associated with significant improvement.

In patients showing an incomplete response, symptoms are reduced, allowing the patient to live a more normal life, but are not eliminated. It should also be noted that stopping drug treatment, even after periods of as much as a year, can precipitate a relapse.

In severe and refractory cases of OCD, neurosurgery may be beneficial (i.e. cingulotomy and capsulotomy). Severe or refractory cases should be referred to clinicians who have advanced training in the treatment of OCD.

Post-traumatic stress disorder (PTSD). The efficacy of both psychological and pharmacological therapy in PTSD is less well established than in other anxiety disorders. The factors determining treatment outcome are not fully understood, but appear to include:

- the nature of the traumatic event
- the response to the trauma
- the interval between the trauma and the start of treatment.

In uncomplicated cases, systematic desensitization (involving exposure in imagination) and relaxation therapies can be useful in reducing arousal and avoidance behavior. Cognitive restructuring therapy may also be beneficial by encouraging the patient to explore the nature of the traumatic event and their response to it. The aim in this case is to reduce the sense of threat and vulnerability.

Among the pharmacological options, tricyclic antidepressants and MAO inhibitors have been most widely studied. These may be useful for the long-term control of symptoms. Efficacy has been established for some of the SSRIs and these may well become the drug treatments of choice for PTSD.

Special populations

Recent guidelines on the pharmacological treatment of anxiety disorders from the British Association for Psychopharmacology contain a number of recommendations for treating:

- children and adolescents
- elderly people
- patients with epilepsy or cardiac problems
- pregnant and breastfeeding women.

Children and adolescents. As some anxiety disorders begin in adolescence, many young people suffer from distressing and intrusive anxiety symptoms. Nevertheless, few controlled

> **Key points – general management**
>
> - Most anxiety conditions are best managed by a combination of psychological and pharmacological therapies.
> - Pure generalized anxiety disorder (GAD), uncomplicated by depression, often goes unrecognized; even when diagnosed, such patients tend to be inadequately treated.
> - Some patients with GAD respond to psychological intervention alone. For others, drug therapy with benzodiazepines, buspirone, antidepressants or β-blockers may be helpful.
> - In all but the mildest cases of panic disorder, drug therapy should be considered, with the aim of controlling rather than curing symptoms.
> - Selective serotonin-reuptake inhibitors are becoming the drug treatment of choice in many anxiety disorders.

trials have been carried out in this population. The balance of risks and benefits for treatment is regarded as unfavorable in depressed adolescents, but more positive in anxious patients as the benefits of therapy appear to be greater and the risk of suicidal features is lower. Nevertheless, close monitoring is needed. Drug treatment may be better reserved for more severely ill patients who are unresponsive to non-drug management.

The elderly. It is often not appreciated that the elderly may experience quite severe anxiety symptoms, either as a worsening of pre-existing anxiety states or as new-onset symptoms in old age. SSRIs or venlafaxine are often effective, but adverse effects, including drug interactions, may be more marked than in younger individuals.

Patients with epilepsy. Most antidepressants lower the seizure threshold; SSRIs present the least risk. Pharmacokinetic interactions are common between antidepressants and many anticonvulsant medications, so the prescriber's vigilance must be high both in the selection of medication and its use. In contrast, benzodiazepines have useful anticonvulsant properties, although tolerance may supervene.

Patients with cardiac problems. TCAs should be avoided as they have significant cardiotoxic effects. SSRIs, on the other hand, are relatively well tolerated and may even have beneficial effects on platelet function. Venlafaxine should be avoided.

Pregnant and breastfeeding women. TCAs and fluoxetine are reasonably safe during pregnancy, and may be needed if relapse threatens after withdrawing medication when a patient becomes pregnant. The drawbacks of benzodiazepines are well known if prescribed around the time of labor.

Paroxetine and sertraline do not cross into the milk during breastfeeding, but citalopram and fluoxetine appear in appreciable levels and should therefore be avoided. Excessively sedating compounds should also be avoided.

Key references

Uhde TW. The anxiety disorders. In: Kryger MH, Roth T, Dement W, eds. *Principles and Practice of Sleep Medicine,* 3rd edn. Philadelphia: WB Saunders, 2000:1123–39.

Weisberg RB, Bruce SE, Machan JT et al. Nonpsychiatric illness among primary care patients with trauma histories and posttraumatic stress disorder. *Psychiatr Serv* 2002;53: 848–54.

Wittchen HU, Kessler RC, Beesdo K et al. Generalized anxiety and depression in primary care: prevalence, recognition, and management. *J Clin Psychiatry* 2002;63(suppl 8):24–34.

Yeragani VK, Radhakrishna RK, Tancer M, Uhde TW. Nonlinear measures of respiration: respiratory irregularity and increased chaos of respiration in patients with panic disorder. *Neuropsychobiology* 2002;46:111–20.

As described in the previous chapter, psychological treatments have an important place in the management of all forms of anxiety disorder. Many of these treatments can be provided in the primary care setting. Others, however, require specialized training and are therefore best provided by a psychiatrist, a clinical psychologist or the community psychiatric services.

Counseling

Counseling can be defined as a 'talking therapy', which aims to ease a person's discomfort, pain, distress or impaired performance. People seeking counseling are regarded as 'clients requiring a service', rather than as patients needing help. Counselors need such skills as the ability to listen to and empathize with the client, and to reflect back what they perceive the client is saying.

Counseling may be:

- non-directive, in which the client is in control of what is discussed in the sessions
- directive, in which specific anxiety-provoking issues in the client's life are identified, and the client is encouraged to face up to them, for example by altering their lifestyle or attitudes.

Such counseling can be undertaken by the family physician or by specially trained counselors. In England and Wales, for example, about one-third of practices employ counselors. Guidelines for the employment of counselors in primary care have been published by the British Association for Counselling and Psychotherapy (see page 81).

Psychotherapy. In focal psychotherapy, the therapist selects a specific topic, and sets an agenda and time limit at the start of treatment. The client is encouraged to talk freely, but the therapist may interrupt to reveal a deeper meaning that the client may not have previously recognized or accepted.

Behavioral therapy

Behavioral therapy appears to be the most effective treatment for phobic disorders. It is also useful in the management of panic disorder without agoraphobia, obsessive–compulsive disorder (OCD), generalized anxiety disorder (GAD) and post-traumatic stress disorder (PTSD).

The most common form of behavioral therapy is exposure to the anxiety-provoking stimulus. Patients are repeatedly exposed to the stimulus until anxiety or panic-like symptoms subside. The systematic desensitization technique described in the previous chapter is an extension of this approach.

Exposure therapy involves five key steps by the patient.
• Commitment to work with the physician or therapist (a written contract is sometimes helpful).
• Writing down specific goals (e.g. control of a specific symptom) that are revised as necessary during treatment.
• Identification of the sensations experienced during symptomatic periods.
• Tackling these sensations with a variety of anxiety management approaches, such as breathing exercises, relaxation techniques and coping strategies.
• Keeping a diary of exposure to the stimulus and its consequences (Figure 6.1).

Plans for future sessions should be made or modified in the light of the experience gained during each session. Patients are normally reviewed 1, 3, 6 and 12 months after completing treatment.

Day/date	Morning	Afternoon	Evening	Night
Sunday	Stayed in	Went to neighbors	Went shopping with husband	Slept well
Monday	Went with friend to gym	Watched tennis on TV	Did ironing	Poor sleep
Tuesday	Had panic attack in garden	Stayed at home	Went to pub with husband	Woke at 4am with panic
Wednesday	Saw GP in surgery; dose of drug upped	Felt sleepy	More relaxed	Slept well
Thursday	Minor panic attack at home; lasted 10 minutes	Felt better	Went shopping with mother	Deep sleep
Friday	Felt quite well	Walked down road on my own	A bit tense	Poor sleep
Saturday	More confident	Mother visited; coped well	OK	Slept well

Overall impression: I think I am better: reduction of 1 on 10-point scale

Figure 6.1 An example of a weekly diary card of a female agoraphobic patient with panics.

Most patients can be treated on an outpatient basis; fewer than 10% require hospitalization. Some patients are effectively treated (i.e. there is total control or elimination of symptoms) after only one or two sessions, but in most cases 4–20 sessions are required. In one specialist unit, patients with OCD required an average of 15 hours' exposure, compared with 10 hours for agoraphobic patients and 5 hours for patients with specific phobias.

Exposure therapy has been reported to produce response rates of at least 66% in patients with agoraphobia, 75–85% in patients with OCD, and up to 90% in patients with specific phobias. Evidence suggests that the improvements are maintained for several years after stopping treatment. A minority of patients do not respond to exposure. This will usually be apparent within the first 2 weeks of treatment, and indicates that treatment should be stopped.

Assertiveness training is sometimes used to enable the patient to respond to interpersonal situations in ways that were previously inhibited by anxiety. Various approaches are used, including role-play and systematic desensitization, to allow the client to express their emotions without anxiety.

Cognitive therapy

Often linked with behavioral therapy, cognitive therapy involves identification of the causes of anxious thinking (i.e. illogical ideas or automatic false notions) and the adoption of more logical (i.e. correct or accurate) ways of thinking. Table 6.1 outlines the approaches used in the management of anxiety. Cognitive therapy has been

TABLE 6.1

Cognitive therapy strategies in the management of anxiety

- Education about the origins of panic symptoms
- Recognition that fear of symptoms can lead to further anxiety, and hence to further symptoms
- Habituation to symptoms such as palpitations or dizziness
- Reversal of the tendency to misinterpret the consequences of symptoms (e.g. loss of control, serious illness)

reported to be more effective than other forms of psychological therapy in the treatment of GAD. However, it requires specialized training, and may therefore not be readily available.

Relaxation techniques

Relaxation training is a useful self-help technique, particularly in patients with GAD. One approach is to teach the client to relax progressively by alternately tensing and relaxing groups of muscles while sitting or lying in a comfortable position. The client then practices doing this more quickly and ultimately learns to apply the technique during daily activities and when feeling anxious.

Biofeedback or meditation techniques may also be useful.

Key points – psychological treatment

- Psychological treatments include psychotherapy, behavioral therapy, cognitive therapy and relaxation techniques.
- In psychotherapy, the client is encouraged to talk freely, but the therapist may intervene to reveal a deeper meaning that has gone unrecognized by the client.
- The most effective treatment for phobic disorders and obsessive–compulsive disorder appears to be behavioral therapy, which generally involves systematic desensitization to the anxiety-provoking stimulus.
- Cognitive therapy may be more effective than other forms of psychological therapy in the treatment of generalized anxiety disorder.

Key reference

Himle JA, Fischer DJ,
Van Etten ML et al. Group
behavioral therapy for adolescents
with tic-related and non-tic-related
obsessive–compulsive disorder.
Depress Anxiety 2003;17:73–7.

Although the drug treatments outlined in Chapter 5 are useful adjuncts to psychological therapy, it should be borne in mind that they relieve symptoms but do not necessarily correct the underlying causes of anxiety. Therefore, a careful assessment of the benefits and risks of pharmacological treatment is necessary. Table 7.1 shows recommendations for the pharmacological treatment of anxiety disorders, while members of each of the main drug classes are listed in Table 7.2.

Benzodiazepines

Benzodiazepines such as clonazepam, alprazolam, lorazepam and diazepam are the most widely used anxiolytic drugs. They act by binding to γ-aminobutyric acid (GABA) receptors, thus enhancing the inhibitory effect of GABA on serotonergic or noradrenergic neurotransmission.

Benzodiazepines have a rapid onset of action, and may produce a mild elevation of mood. Controlled trials have shown that they are effective during short-term treatment (up to 4 weeks), but their beneficial effect appears to be limited; about half of the observed improvement appears to be due to placebo effects.

The efficacy of benzodiazepines during long-term use is less well established. However, some patients may benefit from long-term treatment to prevent a recurrence of anxiety, rather than to control symptoms.

Benzodiazepines are associated with a number of potential problems, including adverse events and the risk of dependence (Table 7.3). Dizziness and ataxia, together with

TABLE 7.1

Recommendations for pharmacological treatment of anxiety disorders (based on guidelines produced by the World Federation of Societies of Biological Psychiatry)

Disorder	First-line agents	Second-line agents	Third-line agents
Generalized anxiety disorder	Venlafaxine SSRIs	Imipramine Buspirone	Unclear
Panic disorder	SSRIs (TCAs)	Benzodiazepines Phenelzine	Moclobemide Nefazodone Valproate Ondansetron
Social anxiety disorder	SSRIs	Phenelzine Moclobemide Benzodiazepines	Venlafaxine Nefazodone Gabapentin Pregabalin
Obsessive–compulsive disorder	SSRIs	Clomipramine	Augmentation with haloperidol, risperidone (or lithium)
Post-traumatic stress disorder	SSRIs	Amitriptyline Imipramine Phenelzine	Unclear

SSRIs, selective serotonin-reuptake inhibitors; TCAs, tricyclic antidepressants.

Source: Based on guidelines published in Bandelow B, Zohar J, Hollander E et al. World Federation of Societies of Biological Psychiatry (WFSBP) guidelines for the pharmacological treatment of anxiety, obsessive–compulsive and post-traumatic stress disorders. *World J Biol Psychiatry* 2002;3:171–9.

psychomotor impairment, can lead to the risk of falls and other accidents at home (particularly in senior citizens) or at work. Similarly, psychomotor impairment has been shown to produce a measurable deterioration in driving skills.

TABLE 7.2

Some members of the principal drug classes used in the management of anxiety disorders

Benzodiazepines
Diazepam
Alprazolam
Clonazepam
Chlordiazepoxide
Lorazepam
Oxazepam

Tricyclic antidepressants
Clomipramine
Imipramine

Selective serotonin-reuptake inhibitors
Paroxetine
Fluoxetine
Sertraline
Citalopram and escitalopram

Selective norepinephrine- and serotonin-reuptake inhibitors
Venlafaxine

Monoamine oxidase inhibitors
Phenelzine
Moclobemide

β-blockers
Propranolol

Sedation occurs in up to 30% of patients, depending on the dose and the drug used; older patients are more sensitive to the sedative effects of benzodiazepines than younger ones.

TABLE 7.3

Potential problems associated with benzodiazepines

Adverse events

Somatic

- – dizziness and ataxia
- – weight gain
- – rash
- – menstrual disturbances

Psychological

- – drowsiness
- – paradoxical anxiety or hostility

Psychomotor

- – impaired attention or coordination
- – development of tolerance to benzodiazepine effect

Cognitive

- – amnesia
- – disrupted consolidation of learning
- – poor subjective memory

Drug interactions

Interactions with other CNS depressants, particularly alcohol

Dependence and abuse

Rebound

Low-dose dependence

High-dose dependence

Abuse, common in association with alcohol or opioids

In addition, physical dependence can develop, even with normal therapeutic regimens. Such dependence is associated with a withdrawal syndrome.

Symptoms of withdrawal include:
- anxiety
- insomnia
- shakiness
- perceptual hypersensitivity
- tremor
- nausea and loss of appetite
- impaired concentration
- headaches and dizziness
- lethargy and tiredness.

Symptoms typically occur within 2 days of stopping a benzodiazepine with a medium duration of action, and 5–10 days after stopping a long-acting agent. They usually subside within a few weeks. Transient rebound phenomena (recurrence of symptoms at a more severe level than before treatment) may also occur when treatment is stopped. The abuse potential of benzodiazepines (e.g. by polydrug abusers) should be carefully evaluated and taken into consideration.

Recognition of the potential adverse events associated with benzodiazepines has led to the development of guidelines for their use in a number of countries. In general, short-term use, preferably with long-acting agents, appears to be appropriate in patients with anxiety disorders. Indeed, such treatment may be justifiable economically as well as clinically, by reducing the financial costs associated with lost productivity among anxious patients. Long-term use and high dosage should, however, be avoided wherever possible.

Tricyclic antidepressants
Tricyclic antidepressants such as imipramine and clomipramine act by inhibiting the reuptake of norepinephrine and serotonin at presynaptic nerve endings. These drugs have

been shown to be effective in panic disorder, generalized anxiety disorder (GAD) and obsessive–compulsive disorder (OCD). However, uncontrolled studies suggest that they are ineffective in patients with social anxiety disorder.

Adverse events associated with tricyclic antidepressants include drowsiness and antimuscarinic effects such as dry mouth, constipation and urinary retention. More seriously, arrhythmias and heart block have occasionally been reported. These cardiovascular effects make overdoses potentially fatal.

Selective serotonin-reuptake inhibitors

There is an increasing trend towards the use of selective serotonin-reuptake inhibitors (SSRIs) in patients with panic disorder. Other indications include GAD, social anxiety disorder, OCD and post-traumatic stress disorder (PTSD).

Drugs that have been studied in clinical trials include paroxetine, fluoxetine and fluvoxamine. A recent meta-analysis of 27 published trials found that SSRIs were significantly more effective than either imipramine or alprazolam, even when high doses of the comparator drugs were used.

SSRIs and the tricyclic antidepressant clomipramine are the current drugs of choice in the treatment of OCD. SSRIs are usually less sedative than tricyclic antidepressants and produce fewer antimuscarinic and cardiovascular effects. Their principal adverse effects are dose-related nausea, vomiting and diarrhea, and sexual dysfunction. This favorable adverse-event profile is largely responsible for the increasing use of these agents in the treatment of anxiety disorders and OCD, as well as in the original indication of depression.

71

Selective norepinephrine- and serotonin-reuptake inhibitors

Venlafaxine has been demonstrated to be effective in the treatment of GAD. It is licensed for this purpose in some countries, including the USA.

Monoamine oxidase inhibitors

Monoamine oxidase (MAO) inhibitors, such as phenelzine, have been shown to be effective in patients with social anxiety disorder and phobic anxiety with depression. However, postural hypotension can be troublesome, and dietary and drug interactions are potentially lethal. In Europe, the selective reversible inhibitor moclobemide, which is well tolerated, is generally preferred.

β-blockers

β-blockers are used in the treatment of GAD and other anxiety disorders when physical symptoms are prominent. Similarly, they may be useful in patients with social anxiety disorder who have a fear of public speaking, vomiting or urinary or fecal incontinence. Low doses are used and side effects are usually minimal.

Buspirone

Buspirone, an agent that acts as a partial agonist at 5-HT_{1A} receptors, lessens anxiety in some patients with GAD. However, the onset of improvement is slower than with benzodiazepines, and may be less marked. Although controversial, there is some evidence that patients previously treated with benzodiazepines may respond less well to buspirone and experience more adverse effects.

The adverse events associated with buspirone appear to be less common and less severe than those associated with

> **Key points – pharmacological treatment**
>
> • Careful assessment of the benefits and risks of pharmacotherapy is essential in all cases.
> • Benzodiazepines are the most widely used anxiolytic drugs. They are effective for short-term treatment.
> • Adverse events associated with benzodiazepines include psychomotor impairment, dizziness, ataxia and sedation. There is also a risk of dependence.
> • Tricyclic antidepressants are effective in treating panic disorder, generalized anxiety disorder (GAD) and obsessive–compulsive disorder (OCD), but overdoses are potentially fatal.
> • The favorable adverse-event profile of selective serotonin-reuptake inhibitors is largely responsible for their increasing use in GAD, panic disorder and OCD, in addition to the original indication of depression.
> • Herbal preparations, such as valerian, and homeopathic remedies may be tried by some patients.

benzodiazepines. The principal adverse events are dizziness, nausea and headache; these can lead to discontinuation in up to 20% of patients. Buspirone does not appear to induce much sedation or to result in dependence, and withdrawal does not lead to rebound symptoms. Abuse is rarely reported.

Atypical antipsychotics

Some patients with anxiety disorders, particularly those with OCD or panic disorder, may have incomplete or partial responses to one or more traditional anti-anxiety or antidepressant medications. Preliminary evidence suggests that the addition of atypical antipsychotic medications to the drug regimen may provide marked therapeutic benefits.

Although atypical antipsychotics produce fewer neurological complications (such as tardive dyskinesia) than traditional antipsychotic compounds (e.g. haloperidol), caution should be exercised in the long-term administration of these agents to patients with non-psychotic disorders. The long-term safety or the risk of extrapyramidal symptoms when using these agents in the treatment of anxiety disorders has not been established. In addition, as a class, atypical antipsychotics have been associated with clinically relevant weight gain, increased triglyceride and cholesterol blood levels, and diabetes.

As a general rule, these agents should be employed by a person with expertise in psychopharmacology and for the treatment of patients who do not respond to traditional anti-anxiety agents.

Other drugs

A wide range of other drugs may be used in some patients. For example, sedative antihistamines such as hydroxyzine are still favored in some European countries because they are non-addictive. Herbal preparations such as valerian are quite popular, and some patients resort to homeopathic remedies.

Recent guidelines

In 2005, the British Association for Psychopharmacology published evidence-based guidelines for the pharmacological treatment of anxiety disorders. For each disorder, the guidelines cover acute and long-term treatment, relapse prevention, drug treatments that enhance the efficacy of psychological therapy and treatments that are effective in non-responsive patients (see Appendix, pages 91–5). The guidelines are based on data from placebo-controlled trials, and are intended to aid clinical decision-making in primary and secondary care.

Key references

Baldwin DS, Anderson IM, Nutt DJ et al. Evidence-based guidelines for the pharmacological treatment of anxiety disorders: recommendations from the British Association for Psycho-pharmacology. *J Psychopharmacol* 2005;19:567-96.

Fallon BA, Liebowitz MR, Campeas R et al. Intravenous clomipramine for obsessive–compulsive disorder refractory to oral clomipramine: a placebo-controlled study. *Arch Gen Psychiatry* 1998;55:918–24.

Kochan LD, Qureshi AI, Fallon BA. Therapeutic approaches to the treatment of refractory obsessive–compulsive disorder. *Curr Psychiatry Rep* 2000;2:327–34.

McDonough M, Kennedy N. Pharmacological management of obsessive–compulsive disorder: a review for clinicians. *Harv Rev Psychiatry* 2002;10:127–37.

Sramek JJ, Zarotsky V, Cutler NR. Generalised anxiety disorder: treatment options. *Drugs* 2002;62: 1635–48.

The neurosciences have developed enormously over the past few decades, although much remains to be clarified. So far, these advances have provided only tantalizing glimpses of the mechanisms that may go awry in various psychiatric conditions.

Molecular neurobiology has revolutionized our thinking about the brain and increased our appreciation of the complex interplay of neurobiological and neuroendocrine substrates that mediate anxiety, stress, arousal, alarm, startle response and related biological functions in humans. At every level, from the functioning of the brain as a processing 'black box', to pathways, neurons, synapses, receptors and other microstructures, each day brings exciting new discoveries.

The advent of neuroimaging has enabled the fine structure of the brain to be depicted in the living human, and the roles of these structures are being worked out using various types of functional neuroimaging. Monitoring of drug effects at the receptor level is also now possible in the living brain. It is inevitable that such advances will impact on our understanding of anxiety, panic and phobias. First, the mechanisms of normal anxiety and fear will be further clarified by identifying the structures and pathways in the brain that subserve these mechanisms. For example, it should become possible to trace the pathways by which a fear-inducing stimulus is processed by following the activation of various parts of the brain. Second, the abnormalities in the brain associated with pathological anxiety and panic will be pinpointed. As a corollary, the processes accompanying successful treatment, both psychological and pharmacological, will be determined.

So far, we have concentrated on the mechanisms underlying symptoms and signs of anxiety and panic. The etiologic factors – genetic, developmental, environmental, psychological, social and so on – will also be clarified. We predict that the most fascinating area will be that of interactions. How does a genetic predisposition express itself? What are the protective factors that prevent panic attacks from being switched on or becoming self-perpetuating? Perhaps those at risk can be identified in some way and preventive measures instituted.

Because neurobiology is currently in a growth spurt, it is easiest to envisage advances in biological treatments. As neuroreceptors are identified and their structure detailed, highly selective drugs could be developed to alter the function of these receptors. It is probably too simplistic, however, to predict that a 'magic bullet' will be found that will change an anxious, panicky individual into one whose repertoire of emotions does not include anxiety. Rather, newer medications with superior risk:benefit ratios are likely to be developed, characterized by rapid onset of action, few side effects, greater therapeutic specificity and no addiction liability.

In parallel, our psychological techniques will become increasingly refined. Rather than merely combating unpleasant or intolerable emotions, these techniques will seek the cognitive abnormalities that accompany and possibly underlie these pathological emotions. The complexities of some of our current psychotherapies, both psychodynamic and cognitive–behavioral, will be clarified. We predict that these apparently very different therapies, based on very different theoretical constructs, will turn out to have many features in common, not least of which will be the doctor–patient or therapist–client relationship.

The next step will be to combine the most useful elements of pharmacological and psychological therapies in order to develop the most efficacious treatments. The components of such combinations and their sequence of use will need careful evaluation. Also, the individuality of each patient must not be overlooked, so that predictive factors for response can be established and applied optimally in each case.

It is important to set the patient or client into his or her psychosocial context to optimize treatment. For example, a judicious mixture of drug and non-drug treatments may help an individual with a phobia of speaking in public. Giving advice about career feasibility goals is also helpful and often essential.

Meanwhile, the best use must be made of our current knowledge and therapeutic techniques. Patients with anxiety, panic and phobias can be greatly helped both symptomatically and behaviorally, and a substantial proportion can resume effective personal, social and occupational functioning. Half-hearted administration of tranquilizers or referral to an inexperienced counselor is not only ineffective, but may also leave the patient or client worse off. This type of outcome should already be a thing of the past.

Key references

Bandelow B, Zohar J, Hollander E et al. World Federation of Societies of Biological Psychiatry (WFSBP) guidelines for the pharmacological treatment of anxiety, obsessive–compulsive and post-traumatic stress disorders. *World J Biol Psychiatry* 2002;3:171–99.

Hoehn-Saric R. Generalised anxiety disorder: guidelines for diagnosis and treatment. *CNS Drugs* 1998; 9:85–98.

Mendlowicz MV, Stein MB. Quality of life in individuals with anxiety disorders. *Am J Psychiatry* 2000;157:669–82.

Nutt D, Ballenger J (eds). *Anxiety Disorders*. Malden, Massachusetts: Blackwell Science, 2003.

Wittchen HU. Generalized anxiety disorder: prevalence, burden, and cost to society. *Depress Anxiety* 2002;16:162–71.

Useful addresses

USA

American Academy of Child and Adolescent Psychiatry
3615 Wisconsin Avenue, NW
Washington, DC 20016-3007
Tel: +1 202 966 7300
Fax: +1 202 966 2891
www.aacap.org

American Psychiatric Association
1000 Wilson Boulevard
Suite 1825, Arlington
VA 22209-3901
Tel: +1 703 907 7300
apa@psych.org
www.psych.org

American Psychiatric Nurses Association
1555 Wilson Boulevard
Suite 602, Arlington, VA 22209
Toll free: 1 866 243 2443
Fax: +1 703 243 3390
www.apna.org

American Psychological Association
750 First Street, NE
Washington, DC 20002-4242
Tel: +1 202 336 5500
Toll free: 1 800 374 2721
www.apa.org

American Psychotherapy Association
2750 E. Sunshine Street
Springfield, MO 65804
Tel: 1 800 205 9165
Fax: +1 417 823 9959
www.americanpsychotherapy.com

Anxiety Disorders Association of America
8730 Georgia Avenue, Suite 600
Silver Spring, MD 20910
Tel: +1 240 485 1001
Fax: +1 240 485 1035
www.adaa.org

National Alliance on Mental Illness
Colonial Place Three
2107 Wilson Boulevard, Suite 300
Arlington, VA 22201-3042
Tel: +1 703 524 7600
Fax: +1 703 524 9094
Helpline: 1 800 950 6264
www.nami.org

National Institute of Mental Health
6001 Executive Boulevard
Room 8184, MSC 9663
Bethesda, MD 20892-9663
Tel: +1 301 443 4513
Toll free: 1 866 615 6464
nimhinfo@nih.gov
www.nimh.nih.gov

Sidran Institute
(helps people understand, and
treat trauma and dissociation)
200 E Joppa Road, Suite 207
Towson, MD 21286
Tel: +1 410 825 8888
Fax: +1 410 337 0747
help@sidran.org (to contact a
trauma resource specialist)
www.sidran.org

Other useful US websites
www.anxietycoach.com
www.anxietypanicattack.com
www.anxietypanicsupport.com
www.ncptsd.va.gov

UK
**British Association for Behavioural
and Cognitive Psychotherapies**
The Globe Centre, PO Box 9
Accrington BB5 0XB
Tel: +44 (0)1254 875277
Fax: +44 (0)1254 239114
babcp@babcp.com
www.babcp.org.uk

**British Association for Counselling
and Psychotherapy**
BACP House
35–37 Albert Street, Rugby
Warwickshire CV21 2SG
Tel: 0870 443 5252
Fax: 0870 443 5161
bacp@bacp.co.uk
www.bacp.co.uk

**British Association for
Psychopharmacology**
BAP Office, 36 Cambridge Place
Hills Road, Cambridge CB2 1NS
Tel: +44 (0)1223 358395
www.bap.org.uk

The British Psychological Society
St Andrews House
48 Princess Road East
Leicester LE1 7DR
Tel: +44 (0)116 254 9568
Fax: +44 (0)116 247 0787
enquiry@bps.org.uk
www.bps.org.uk

The Child Death Helpline
Child Death Helpline Dept
Great Ormond Street Hospital
London WC1N 3JH
Tel: +44 (0)20 7813 8551
Helpline: 0800 282986
(Mon–Fri 10 AM–1 PM,
Wed 1–4 PM, evenings 7–10 PM)
www.childdeathhelpline.org.uk

The Compassionate Friends
(support and encouragement after
the death of a child)
53 North Street, Bristol BS3 1EN
Tel: 0845 120 3785
Helpline: 0845 123 2304
(10 AM–4 PM/6.30–10.30 PM)
info@tcf.org.uk
www.tcf.org.uk

Cruse Bereavement Care
(support and information
following bereavement)
Cruse House, 126 Sheen Road
Richmond, Surrey TW9 1UR
Tel: +44 (0)20 8939 9530
Helpline: 0870 167 1677
helpline@crusebereavementcare.
org.uk
www.crusebereavementcare.
org.uk

First Steps to Freedom
(advice on overcoming anxiety
disorders and on tranquilizer
withdrawal)
1 Taylor Close, Kenilworth
Warwickshire CV8 2LW
Tel/fax: +44 (0)1926 864473
Helpline: 0845 120 2916
(7 days a week 10 AM–10 PM)
first.steps@btconnect.com
www.first-steps.org

Mind (The Mental Health Charity)
15–19 Broadway
London E15 4BQ
Tel: +44 (0)20 8519 2122
Fax: +44 (0)20 8522 1725
Mind*info*Line: 0845 766 0163
(Mon–Fri 9.15 AM–5.15 PM)
contact@mind.org.uk
www.mind.org.uk

National Phobics Society
Zion Community Resource
Centre, 339 Stretford Road
Hulme, Manchester M15 4ZY
Tel: 0870 122 2325
Fax: +44 (0)161 226 7727
info@phobics-society.org.uk
www.phobics-society.org.uk

No Panic
(support for sufferers of panic
attacks, phobias, OCD, GAD, and
for tranquilizer withdrawal)
93 Brands Farm Way
Telford, Shropshire TF3 2JQ
Tel: +44 (0)1952 590005
Helpline: 0808 808 0545
(7 days a week 10 AM–10 PM)
Fax: +44 (0)1952 270 962
ceo@nopanic.org.uk
www.nopanic.org.uk

Primhe
Primary Care Mental Health &
Education, Unit 6
2a Laurel Avenue, Twickenham
Middlesex TW1 4JA
Tel: +44 (0)20 8891 6593
admin@primhe.org
www.primhe.org

The Royal College of Psychiatrists
17 Belgrave Square
London SW1X 8PG
Tel: +44 (0)20 7235 2351
Fax: +44 (0)20 7245 1231
rcpsych@rcpsych.ac.uk
www.rcpsych.ac.uk

Scottish Association for
Mental Health
Cumbrae House
15 Carlton Court
Glasgow G5 9JP
Tel: +44 (0)141 568 7000
enquire@samh.org.uk
www.samh.org.uk

SANE & SANELINE
(information, support and
research on all mental illnesses)
1st Floor, Cityside House
40 Adler Street, London E1 1EE
Tel: +44 (0)20 7375 1002
Fax: +44 (0)20 7375 2162
Helpline: 0845 767 8000
(Mon–Fri 12 noon–11 PM;
Sat/Sun 12 noon–6 PM)
www.sane.org.uk

The Stress Management Society
PO Box 193, Harrow
Middlesex HA1 3ZE
Tel: 0870 199 3260
info@stress.org.uk
www.stress.org.uk

Triumph Over Phobia (TOP UK)
(network of self-help groups for
people with phobia or OCD)
PO Box 3760, Bath BA2 4WY
Tel: 0845 600 9601
info@triumphoverphobia.org.uk
www.triumphoverphobia.com

Why Me?
(advice and support for sufferers
of anxiety and related disorders)
6 Thorney Close, Fareham
Hampshire PO14 3AF
Helpline: +44 (0)1329 312997
(Mon–Fri 9 AM–6 PM)

Other useful UK websites
www.anxietycare.org.uk
www.nomorepanic.co.uk

International
Anxiety Disorders Alliance
60–62 Victoria Road
Gladesville, NSW 2111
Tel: +61 (0)2 9879 5351
Helpline: 1 800 626 055
ocd@ada.mentalhealth.asn.au
www.ada.mentalhealth.asn.au

Anxiety Treatment Australia
Floor 1, 140–142 Barkers Road
Hawthorn 3122, Victoria
Tel: +61 (0)3 9819 3671
catherine@socialanxietyassist
.com.au
www.anxietyaustralia.com.au

Association of European
Psychiatrists
5, quai de Paris
F-67000 Strasbourg, France
Tel: +33 (0)3 88 23 99 30
Fax: +33 (0)3 88 35 29 73
aep.strasbourg@wanadoo.fr
www.aep.lu

Collegium Internationale Neuro-
Psychopharmacologicum
1608 17th Avenue South
Nashville, TN 37212, USA
Tel: +1 615 297 3144
Fax: +1 615 385 3174
www.cinp.org

European College of
Neuropsychopharmacology
ECNP Office, PO Box 85410
3508 AK Utrecht
The Netherlands
Tel: +31 (0)30 253 8567
Fax: +31 (0)30 253 8568
secretariat@ecnp.nl
www.ecnp.nl

European Federation of
Psychologists' Associations
EFPA Head Office
Grasmarkt 105/18
B-1000 Brussels, Belgium
Tel: +32 (0)2 503 49 53
Fax: +32 (0)2 503 30 67
www.efpa.be

Global Alliance of Mental Illness
Advocacy Networks
GAMIAN, 308 Seaview Avenue
Staten Island, NY 10305, USA
Tel: +1 718 351 1717
Fax: +1 718 667 8893
www.gamian.org

The International Society for
Affective Disorders
Institute of Psychiatry
King's College London
De Crespigny Park, Denmark Hill
London, SE5 8AF
isad@isad.org.uk
www.isad.org.uk

The International Stress
Management Association
(see UK website for contacts in
other countries)
ISMA UK, PO Box 26
South Petherton TA13 5WY
Tel: +44 (0)7000 780430
stress@isma.org.uk
www.isma.org.uk

Other useful international websites
www.anxietycentre.com (Canada)
www.wpanet.org

Appendix: Caffeine in beverages and medications

TABLE A1

Average caffeine concentration of various beverages

	Caffeine content (mg)
Coffee	
Percolated (7 fluid oz)	140
Drip (7 fluid oz)	115–175
Espresso (1.5–2 fluid oz)	100
Brewed (7 fluid oz)	80–135
Instant (7 fluid oz)	65–100
Brewed decaffeinated (6 fluid oz)	5
Tea	
Iced tea (12 fluid oz)	70
Green tea (6 fluid oz)	35
Instant tea (7 fluid oz)	30
Instant decaffeinated (6 fluid oz)	3
Cola drinks (mg/12 fluid oz)	
Afri Cola	100
Jolt	72
Sugar-Free Mr Pibb	58.8
Pepsi One	55
Tab	46.8
Diet Coca Cola	45
Shasta Cola	44.4
Royal Crown Cola	43.2
Dr Pepper	41
Mr Pibb	40.8
Diet Mr Pibb	40.5

(CONTINUED)

TABLE A1 (CONTINUED)

Average caffeine concentration of various beverages

	Caffeine content (mg)
Pepsi	38.4
Diet RC Cola	36
Diet Rite	36
Coca Cola	34
Canada Dry Cola	30
Cherry Cola	23
Canada Dry Diet Cola	1.2
Non-cola drinks (mg/12 fluid oz or as specified)	
Red Bull (80 mg/8.3 fluid oz)	115.5
Java Water (125 mg/16.9 fluid oz)	88.8
Bawls (67 mg/10 fluid oz)	80
Krank 20 (100 mg/16.9 fluid oz)	71
XTC Power Drink	70
Diet Sun Drop	69
Aqua Blast (90 mg/16.9 fluid oz)	63.9
Dun Drop	63
Josta	58
Kick	57.6
Mountain Dew	55
Kick Citrus	54
KMX	53
Surge	52.5
Mello Yellow	51
Nehi Wild Red	50.1
Battery Energy Drink	46.7
Water Joe (60–70 mg/16.9 fluid oz)	~46.2
Sunkist	41

(CONTINUED)

TABLE A1 (CONTINUED)

Average caffeine concentration of various beverages

	Caffeine content (mg)
Red Flash	40.5
Aqua Java (50–60 mg/16.9 fluid oz)	~39.1
Ruby Red Squirt	39
Aspen	36
Snapple Lemon	31.5
Snapple Peach	31.5
Snapple Raspberry	31.5
A&W Cream Soda	29
Nestea Sweet Iced Tea	26.5
Snapple Green Tea with Lemon	24
Barq's	22.5
A&W Diet Cream Soda	22
Mistic Lemon Tea	18
Mistic Peach Tea	18
Cool Nestea	16.5
Nestea Iced Tea	16.5
Snapple Sweet Tea	12
Diet Cool Nestea	10.5
Fanta Orange	0
Fresca	0
Hires Root Beer	0
Patio Orange	0
Sprite	0
7 UP	0

TABLE A2

Caffeine in medications

	Caffeine content (mg/tablet)
Kirkaffeine	250
Caffedrine	200
Dexatrim	200
EFED II	200
Maximum Strength Awake	200
NoDoz, Maximum Strength	200
Ultra Pep-back	200
Vivarin	200
Quick Pep	150
Awake	100
Cafergot	100
Migralam	100
NoDoz	100
Wigraine	100
Aqua-Ban	~65–100
Arthriten	65
Excedrin	65
Midol Maximum Strength	60
Norgesic Forte	60
Fat Burner	~55
Migrol	50
XS Hangover Relief	50
Amaphen	40
Analor 300	40
Anoquan	40
Butalbital	40

(CONTINUED)

TABLE A2 (CONTINUED)

Caffeine in medications

	Caffeine content (mg/tablet)
Epam	40
Esgic	40
Femcet	40
Fioricet	40
Fiorinal	40
Medigesic	40
Pacaps	40
Tenake capsules	40
Triad	40
Vanquish	33
Goody's X-Strength Headache Powders	32.5
Darvon	32.4
Mido (original and extra strength)	32.4
PC-CAP	32.4
Propoxyphene Compound 65	32.4
SK-65 compound	32.4
Alpha-phed	32
Anacin	32
Beta-phed	32
Cope	32
Gelprin	32
Stanback Headache Powders	32
Codalan (1, 2 & 3)	30
Compal	30
Coryban D	30
DHC Plus	30
Diagesic	30

(CONTINUED)

TABLE A2 (CONTINUED)

Caffeine in medications

	Caffeine content (mg/tablet)
Dristan	30
Korigesic	30
Norgesic	30
Synalgos DC capsules	30
Goody's X-Strength Pain Relief	16.25
Caffeine Mints	~12

Appendix: Evidence-based treatment guidelines

TABLE A3

Clinically available evidence-based treatments for generalized anxiety disorder

	SSRIs	TCAs	BZPs	Others
Acute efficacy	Escitalopram Paroxetine Sertraline	Imipramine	Alprazolam Diazepam	Venlafaxine CBT Buspirone Hydroxyzine Pregabalin Trifluoperazine
Long-term efficacy	Escitalopram Paroxetine	–	–	CBT Venlafaxine
Relapse prevention	Paroxetine Escitalopram	–	–	CBT
Enhances efficacy of psychological treatment	–	–	Diazepam	–

– No published placebo-controlled data available.
BZPs, benzodiazepines; CBT, cognitive–behavioral therapy; SSRIs, selective serotonin-reuptake inhibitors; TCAs, tricyclic antidepressants.

Reproduced with permission of Sage Publications Ltd from Baldwin DS, Anderson IM, Nutt DJ et al. Evidence-based guidelines for the pharmacological treatment of anxiety disorders: recommendations of the British Association for Psychopharmacology. *J Psychopharmacol* 2005;19:567–96. Copyright © 2005 British Association for Psychopharmacology.

TABLE A4

Clinically available evidence-based treatments for panic disorder

	SSRIs	TCAs	BZPs	Others
Acute panic attack	–	–	Alprazolam Lorazepam	–
Acute efficacy	Citalopram Escitalopram Fluoxetine Fluvoxamine Paroxetine Sertraline	Clomipramine Imipramine	Alprazolam Clonazepam Diazepam Lorazepam	CBT Phenelzine Moclobemide* Mirtazapine* Venlafaxine Reboxetine Na valproate
Long-term efficacy	Citalopram Fluoxetine Paroxetine Sertraline	Clomipramine Imipramine	Alprazolam	Moclobemide* CBT
Relapse prevention	Fluoxetine Paroxetine Sertraline	Imipramine	–	CBT
Enhances efficacy of psychological treatment	Paroxetine	Antidepressants[†]	BZPs[†]	Buspirone
After non-response	Paroxetine (prior CBT)	–	–	Pindolol Group CBT

– No published placebo-controlled data available.
*Comparator-controlled study only. [†]Meta-analysis data.
BZPs, benzodiazepines; CBT, cognitive–behavioral therapy; SSRIs, selective serotonin-reuptake inhibitors; TCAs, tricyclic antidepressants.

Reproduced with permission of Sage Publications Ltd from Baldwin DS, Anderson IM, Nutt DJ et al. Evidence-based guidelines for the pharmacological treatment of anxiety disorders: recommendations of the British Association for Psychopharmacology. *J Psychopharmacol* 2005;19:567–96. Copyright © 2005 British Association for Psychopharmacology.

TABLE A5

Clinically available evidence-based treatments for social anxiety disorder

	SSRIs	TCAs	BZPs	Others
Acute efficacy	Escitalopram Fluoxetine Fluvoxamine Paroxetine Sertraline	–	Bromazepam Clonazepam	CBT Phenelzine Moclobemide Venlafaxine Gabapentin Pregabalin Olanzapine
Long-term efficacy	Escitalopram Fluvoxamine Paroxetine Sertraline	–	–	CBT Phenelzine Moclobemide Venlafaxine
Relapse prevention	Escitalopram Paroxetine Sertraline	–	Clonazepam	CBT
Enhances efficacy of psychological treatment	Sertraline	–	–	–

– No published placebo-controlled data available.
BZPs, benzodiazepines; CBT, cognitive–behavioral therapy; SSRIs, selective serotonin-reuptake inhibitors; TCAs, tricyclic antidepressants.

Reproduced with permission of Sage Publications Ltd from Baldwin DS, Anderson IM, Nutt DJ et al. Evidence-based guidelines for the pharmacological treatment of anxiety disorders: recommendations of the British Association for Psychopharmacology. *J Psychopharmacol* 2005;19:567–96. Copyright © 2005 British Association for Psychopharmacology.

TABLE A6

Clinically available evidence-based treatments for obsessive–compulsive disorder

	SSRIs	TCAs	BZPs	Others
Acute efficacy	Citalopram Fluoxetine Fluvoxamine Paroxetine Sertraline	Clomipramine Imipramine	Clonazepam?	CBT
Long-term efficacy	Fluoxetine Sertraline	Clomipramine	–	CBT
Relapse prevention	Fluoxetine Paroxetine Sertraline	–	–	–
Enhances efficacy of psychological treatment	Fluvoxamine	Clomipramine	–	–
After non-response	–	–	Clonazepam	Another SSRI Haloperidol* Risperidone* Quetiapine* Pindolol*

– No published placebo-controlled data available.
*Placebo-controlled augmentation study.
BZPs, benzodiazepines; CBT, cognitive–behavioral therapy; SSRIs, selective serotonin-reuptake inhibitors; TCAs, tricyclic antidepressants.

TABLE A7

Clinically available evidence-based treatments for post-traumatic stress disorder

	SSRIs	TCAs	BZPs	Others
Prevention of PT symptoms?	–	–	–	Hydrocortisone Propranolol Trauma-focused CBT
Acute efficacy	Fluoxetine Paroxetine Sertraline	Amitriptyline Imipramine	Alprazolam	Trauma-focused CBT EMDR Brofaromine Phenelzine Lamotrigine Mirtazapine Venlafaxine
Long-term efficacy	Sertraline	–	–	–
Relapse prevention	Fluoxetine Sertraline	–	–	CBT?
After non-response	–	–	–	Olanzapine* Risperidone*

– No published placebo-controlled data available.
*Placebo-controlled augmentation study.
BZPs, benzodiazepines; CBT, cognitive–behavioral therapy; EMDR, eye movement desensitization and reprocessing; PT, post-traumatic; SSRIs, selective serotonin-reuptake inhibitors; TCAs, tricyclic antidepressants.

Reproduced with permission of Sage Publications Ltd from Baldwin DS, Anderson IM, Nutt DJ et al. Evidence-based guidelines for the pharmacological treatment of anxiety disorders: recommendations of the British Association for Psychopharmacology. *J Psychopharmacol* 2005;19:567–96. Copyright © 2005 British Association for Psychopharmacology.

Index

GAD, generalized anxiety disorder; OCD, obsessive–compulsive disorder; PTSD, post-traumatic stress disorder.